Legal Encroachment on Psychiatric Practice

Stephen Rachlin, *Editor*

NEW DIRECTIONS FOR MENTAL HEALTH SERVICES
H. RICHARD LAMB, *Editor-in-Chief*

Number 25, March 1985

Paperback sourcebooks in
The Jossey-Bass Social and Behavioral Sciences Series

Jossey-Bass Inc., Publishers
San Francisco • Washington • London

Stephen Rachlin (Ed).
Legal Encroachment on Psychiatric Practice.
New Directions for Mental Health Services, no. 25.
San Francisco: Jossey-Bass, 1985.

New Directions for Mental Health Services Series
H. Richard Lamb, *Editor-in-Chief*

New Directions for Mental Health Services (publication number
USPS 493-910) is published quarterly by Jossey-Bass Inc.,
Publishers. Second-class postage rates paid at San Francisco,
California, and at additional mailing offices.

Correspondence:
Subscriptions, single-issue orders, change of address notices, undelivered
copies, and other correspondence should be sent to Subscriptions,
Jossey-Bass Inc., Publishers, 433 California Street, San Francisco
California 94104.

Editorial correspondence should be sent to the Editor-in-Chief,
H. Richard Lamb, Department of Psychiatry and the Behavioral
Sciences, U.S.C. School of Medicine, 1934 Hospital Place,
Los Angeles, California 90033.

Library of Congress Catalogue Card Number LC 84-82374

International Standard Serial Number ISSN 0193-9416

International Standard Book Number ISBN 87589-759-2

Cover art by Willi Baum
Manufactured in the United States of America

Ordering Information

The paperback sourcebooks listed below are published quarterly and can be ordered either by subscription or single-copy.

Subscriptions cost $35.00 per year for institutions, agencies, and libraries. Individuals can subscribe at the special rate of $25.00 per year *if payment is by personal check.* (Note that the full rate of $35.00 applies if payment is by institutional check, even if the subscription is designated for an individual.) Standing orders are accepted. Subscriptions normally begin with the first of the four sourcebooks in the current publication year of the series. When ordering, please indicate if you prefer your subscription to begin with the first issue of the *coming* year.

Single copies are available at $8.95 when payment accompanies order, and *all single-copy orders under $25.00 must include payment.* (California, New Jersey, New York, and Washington, D.C., residents please include appropriate sales tax.) For billed orders, cost per copy is $8.95 plus postage and handling. (Prices subject to change without notice.)

Bulk orders (ten or more copies) of any individual sourcebook are available at the following discounted prices: 10–49 copies, $8.05 each; 50–100 copies, $7.15 each; over 100 copies, *inquire.* Sales tax and postage and handling charges apply as for single copy orders.

To ensure correct and prompt delivery, all orders must give either the *name of an individual* or an *official purchase order number.* Please submit your order as follows:

Subscriptions: specify series and year subscription is to begin.
Single Copies: specify sourcebook code (such as, MHS8) and first two words of title.

Mail orders for United States and Possessions, Latin America, Canada, Japan, Australia, and New Zealand to:
    Jossey-Bass Inc., Publishers
    433 California Street
    San Francisco, California 94104

Mail orders for all other parts of the world to:
    Jossey-Bass Limited
    28 Banner Street
    London EC1Y 8QE

New Directions for Mental Health Services Series
H. Richard Lamb, *Editor-in-Chief*

Contents

Editor's Notes

Another anthology on psychiatry and the law? With so many good books already available on the subject, that was the question I asked when the opportunity to edit this volume was presented. Intrigued by the possibilities of going beyond a discourse on the bare facts into commentary and polemic, I accepted.

We all rather naturally have our ire aroused when outsiders attempt to regulate or otherwise control our professional practice. Certainly, none of us is above scrutiny in this era of accountability, but we tend strongly to believe that our own ethical standards and peer review are sufficient to assure quality patient care. When this conviction is challenged, we often respond angrily. We would do well to remember, however, that many of the legal requirements now upon us developed, in part, because of some very obvious shortcomings in the ways in which treatment was provided in the public sector. While we distinguish that which was the foreseeable result of governmental underfunding of service or an inevitable outcome of the realistic limits of scientific knowledge from deficiences that might be laid at our doorstep, we have not regularly conveyed this message to legislative bodies and the legal system, nor have they always been willing to listen.

In an effort to help change that, I have assembled an outstanding group of practitioners and teachers of forensic psychiatry for this sourcebook. All are involved in the activities of the American Academy of Psychiatry and the Law, the premier medical organization devoted to this particular interface; most also are diplomates of the American Board of Forensic Psychiatry. The authors have all published widely, and most have done prior work in the subjects that they address here. This time, they were asked to give it a different slant—to take the gloves off, as it were.

At the risk of being accused of parochialism, I have chosen only psychiatrists as contributors; two are also attorneys. I made this decision not only because these are the people I know best but also because I believe that, of the mental health professions, we are presently the most intensely involved with medicolegal matters. All this may change in the future. If psychologists, social workers, nurses, and others reach parity of independent practice with psychiatrists, in terms of hospital admitting privileges, full insurance reimbursement for services rendered, or some other level, they, too, will be subjected to the same scrutiny that we now decry.

It was also my conscious choice to limit our focus to issues primarily related to civil law. Although this eliminates from discussion such headline grabbers as the insanity defense, it allows us to pay attention to concerns that are relevant to the day-to-day work of the average clinician.

This is the third *New Directions for Mental Health Services* sourcebook devoted to psychiatry and the law. For further background, the reader is referred to *Coping with the Legal Onslaught* (Halleck, 1979) and *The Mental Health Professional and the Legal System* (Gross and Weinberger, 1982). I am pleased to have the opportunity to present an update current to summer 1984.

Chapter One originated in a series of stimulating discussions that I had with Gutheil and Mills. It sets the tone for what follows by providing an orientation to the differences between the ways in which medical and legal personnel think through their decisions. Included are the logical frameworks, the adversary system, judgmental biases, precedent, and the balance between rights and needs. The fundamental discrepancy between what the law calls *findings* and what science knows as *empiricism* is crucial.

Miller begins Chapter Two by noting that civil commitment cuts across most areas of legal involvement in clinical practice. The impact has been both far-reaching and very visible. The assault on involuntary hospitalization has a number of theoretical bases. In the early days, many health professionals aided the cause, sharing only the hope that conditions for our patients would improve. Activist attorneys interposed their ideology and values without any agreement that those were in any concrete way better than our own. There are signs that the tide of change may have crested.

We have come a long way from the time when admission to a mental hospital was equated with incompetence. In Chapter Three, Sadoff reviews the historical development of the concept of competence, showing how professional standards were raised by increased consciousness of the parameters and contexts in which the question of competence can arise. While we pay much more than lip service to the patient's right to give fully informed consent to proposed procedures, the frontier area lies in determining just how much information must be disclosed. This is as much a matter of ethics as it is of law. Appropriate guidelines are central to implementing the right to treatment, among others, in the interests of patient autonomy.

Of all the class action lawsuits on behalf of the hospitalized mentally ill, the perigee in terms of palatability is the *Rogers* right-to-refuse-treatment case. In Chapter Four, Gutheil dissects this decision of the Supreme Judicial Court of Massachusetts and the earlier rulings that underlie it. He shows that there are many paradoxes between what the courts have said and what we as clinicians know to be true. The ruling is an extreme one, out of step with most other similar litigation, and its full impact has yet to be assessed. Antithetical to *parens patriae* approaches to treatment, it has summoned the pique of many of us. In addition, the legally complicated procedures demanded by the court will be expensive to implement.

Dollars are also relevant to Perr, who gives us an insight into the real-life working of the system of malpractice law in Chapter Five. The author is qualified to poke some fun at attorneys, since he possesses a legal degree. He has been a student of this subject for a number of years, and he shares the benefits of his experience with us. Right now, psychiatrists are not often sued.

This may have to do with the particular nature of our work, which has its own distinct Achilles' heels. For example, we are increasingly being held accountable for the actions and behavior of our patients. The post hoc determinations of dangerousness and suicidality that are now being made are making prevention and risk management increasingly difficult.

In Chapter Six, Mills, who also is trained in law, explores one special area of litigation. Virtually all practicing mental health professionals have heard of the *Tarasoff* case, which gave rise to the so-called duty to warn. Widely quoted, yet almost as often misunderstood, *Tarasoff* imposes the obligation simply to exercise reasonable care to protect potential victims. There are a variety of ways in which this objective can be accomplished. The original decision has not been affirmed in all jurisdictions, but some recent decisions in California may have expanded the scope of our legal obligations. The author's conclusion is as intriguing as it is provocative.

Responsibility to a third party is not precluded by the principle of confidentiality. In Chapter Seven, Bursten shows that each argument in favor of maintaining secrecy can be rebutted. There may not really be any absolutes in our obligation to maintain patients' privacy, for competing societal interests, such as the needs of justice, will always require some exceptions. Will psychiatry's concern for confidentiality stay high, or will it give way to other pressures and requirements? As a concept, is it better thought of as a sword or as a shield?

Material in a medical record has frequently been kept away from the patient whom it involves. As the final example of values in conflict, Schwartz and I look in Chapter Eight at the question of access to charts. This question may turn out to be a tempest in a teapot, fears to the contrary notwithstanding. Much of the activity in this arena has been legislative, not judicial. The little data in the scientific literature about the effect of seeing one's own records have not shown clearly that it is detrimental. We recommend a qualified right of access designed to protect both patients and practitioners.

That the law is well entrenched in matters of mental health and illness is clear. Whether the law is also encroaching upon what we think of as our proper domain is a judgment that the reader is now invited to make.

Stephen Rachlin
Editor

References

Gross, B. H., and Weinberger, L. E. (Eds.). *The Mental Health Professional and the Legal System.* New Directions for Mental Health Services, no. 16. San Francisco: Jossey-Bass, 1982.

Halleck, S. (Ed.). *Coping with the Legal Onslaught.* New Directions for Mental Health Services, no. 4. San Francisco: Jossey-Bass, 1979.

Stephen Rachlin is chairman, Department of Psychiatry and Psychology, Nassau County Medical Center (East Meadow, New York); associate professor of clinical psychiatry, State University of New York at Stony Brook School of Medicine; and special professor of law and psychiatry, Hofstra University School of Law.

*Psychiatry and law often use different models of decision making
to arrive at their respective conclusions. Sometimes, these divergent
models indicate a controversy over fundamental values.*

Differing Conceptual Models in Psychiatry and Law

Thomas G. Gutheil, Stephen Rachlin, Mark J. Mills

*Put most simply, the law can and should be submitted to fundamental
criticism, and such criticism cannot come from the law itself.*
Buchanan, (1979)

When court decisions that affect psychiatric practice appear to be out of step
with clinical principles, psychiatrists are apt to complain that psychiatry is
misunderstood. But, why should one expect the judiciary to know more about
psychiatry than it does about other scientific areas? It is as apparent that the
law sometimes fails to grasp the subtleties of mental health and illness as it is
clear that psychiatrists are often unaware of the nuances of law. After all, both
fields are complex and highly developed, and each requires extensive training
to master. Yet, as the epigraph to this chapter suggests, one learned discipline
may be a useful vantage point from which to examine, even to criticize, the
other.

Conflicting Models

Toward this end, we (Gutheil and Mills, 1982; Rachlin, 1982) have
described some of the conceptual and ideological differences between clinical
and legal models that contribute to interdisciplinary miscomprehension.

S. Rachlin (Ed.). *Legal Encroachment on Psychiatric Practice.* New Directions for
Mental Health Services, no. 25. San Francisco: Jossey-Bass, March 1985.

6

Could it be that the Supreme Court is recognizing that imposition of one system's viewpoint on the other's is creating as many problems as it is solving? Appelbaum (1984) has identified the Court's ostensible intention to limit judicial involvement in the running of institutions. One path to this goal involves the defining of specific procedures deemed adequate to protect rights. For example, in *Youngberg* v. *Romeo* (1982), the Court advocated deference to professional judgment in determination of the circumstances under which substantive constitutional rights could be abridged in the name of treatment exigencies.

While the value of studying the other's viewpoint might seem obvious, the two disciplines have made little effort to do so, probably because each discipline achieves high levels of internal (consensual) validation and because each discipline is insulated from both the data and the conceptual frameworks of the other. Thus, in litigation over the right to refuse treatment (Mills and others, 1983; Chapter Four of this volume), courts have judged antipsychotic medications to be "mind-altering" and "thought-controlling" drugs. The courts' major source of information was polemical legal literature, which proposed pharmacological notions lacking balance, realism, and perspective. Gutheil and Appelbaum (1983) responded to these distortions with a law journal article that reviewed the actual mechanisms of antipsychotic medications. Such publications make empirical data available to attorneys and judges, who tend not to read the clinical literature. In this chapter, we propose to extend previous work by clarifying how the contrasting conceptual models of decision making in psychiatry and law can impede interdisciplinary understanding.

Theoretical Issues

Inductive Versus Deductive. One common starting point in comparisons of law and medicine is the reliance of law on inductive reasoning and of medicine on deductive reasoning. There are exceptions, to be sure, but the distinction is useful for didactic purposes. According to this model, the typical psychiatric method of drawing conclusions is to go from the general to the particular: from the theory, principle, or diagnostic criteria to the individual case with which one is dealing. In contrast, the law begins with the specific case at bar and infers broader principles from it. To illustrate from actual practice, a court may first decide what is just in a specific situation, then base its analysis of the fundamental rights at issue on that decision.

Adversary Versus Ally. Another, often problematic, area involves the centrality of the adversary system in law; in contrast, alliance is central to psychiatry. The essence of law is the disagreement or conflict. If there were no conflict, there would be no case: The very fact that a case is being tried indicates both that disagreement exists and that efforts at compromise have failed. One implication of this central fact is that the outcome must define a winner and a loser; the law is a "zero-sum game" (Gutheil and Magraw, 1984). In contrast, mental health professionals think in terms of collaboration; their job is to take care of those who cannot fend for themselves. There is usually no real conflict as the law defines it, although disagreements are not uncommon.

In court, the adversary process can be quite confusing to the uninitiated. Like true opponents in battle, each side's lawyer fights, as he or she is mandated, to make that side look best. It is not that counsel cannot see or grasp the opposing points. In fact, a traditional law school exercise requires the student to prepare both sides of a case fully and independently. Similarly, the participants in a moot court may not be assigned their client until just before the trial begins. The central issue here is that the lawyer's task is defined as one of presenting a single side of the case. It is this type of background that enables lawyers to represent either side of a given case without conflict.

Legal Versus Clinical Judgment. Another area of conflict involves the concept of judgment. The legal system is founded on the concept of judgment, yet clinical work generally strives to be nonjudgmental. Paradoxically, courts can elect not to judge (that is, not to decide), while clinicians cannot. This paradox requires some explication. Courts enjoy many methods of sidestepping an issue: continuance, appeal, selection of just one part of an issue, even refusal to address the issue at all. For example, the United States Supreme Court, despite a number of opportunities to do so, has repeatedly avoided determining whether there is a constitutional right to refuse treatment (*Mills v. Rogers,* 1982). In contrast, many events in patient care preclude such passivity: Clinicians must often make immediate clinical judgments that brook no delay. In some circumstances, doing nothing is, in and of itself, a decision. Clinicians rarely can wait until a matter becomes "ripe."

Problems of Precedent. Regional precedent is another confusing feature in law. A determination can be made in one jurisdiction, while an adjoining jurisdiction can hold the opposite. In essence, regional precedent establishes rules that hold in one area only. It might be argued that similar psychiatric ideologies display certain patterns and that some of these patterns can be defined regionally. For example, we speak of a "Chicago school." Because of national vehicles and organizations for communication and sharing of ideas, much of the regionalism in both disciplines is breaking down. In the short run, however, startling ideological disparities can still exist between geographically adjacent regions.

Rights Versus Needs. Consider also the balance between rights and needs. As Rachlin (1975, p. 99) stated nearly a decade ago, "When rights are not consonant with needs, they lose much of their value." Clinicians are concerned primarily with the individual patient's needs. Treatment aims at the patient's welfare, and the most important measure is the actual outcome. In contrast, courts are often more concerned with process—"due process"—than with outcome. In addition, courts tend to stress perceived rights, which represent an impersonal normative or collective concept. Thus, in a class action lawsuit, all individuals similarly situated seek a remedy as a group. This

8

approach confuses clinicians, whose usual focus is the individual patient's needs. Of course, in other circumstances, the judiciary pays significant attention to individuals as well. The classic examples of the acrimony that this aspect of disparate perceptions can create involve involuntary hospitalization (Chapter Two in this volume) and the right to refuse treatment (Chapter Four in this volume).

Legal Findings and Scientific Empiricism

One of the most revealing differences in the terminology of psychiatry and law is captured in their use of the word findings. In psychiatry, the term points to empirical observations gleaned from conversation with and direct observation of patients. Thus, the psychiatrists' "findings" can include the patient's disheveled appearance—a direct observation—as well as the patient's inability to abstract the meaning of proverbs—an assessment of verbal responses to the provocative test of asking for interpretations. Both "findings" represent raw data that the psychiatrist would join with other data against the backdrop of possible disease entities in order to make a tentative diagnosis. The diagnosis represents the conclusion of the processing of the original "findings."

In contrast, the term *findings* in law most often refers to the final outcome, that is, to the conclusion of decision that caps the result. Thus, when a judge says, "We find the defendant guilty," he or she means that the raw data supplied by the testimony of witnesses and experts, measured against the backdrop of precedent and case law, leads to a final decision or conclusion about guilt or liability.

Findings Versus Reality. One important latent aspect of this critical difference in the ways in which law and psychiatry conceive of findings is that the findings in psychiatric (as in other scientific) explorations preexist the procedure designed to elicit them. That is, the patient's inability to abstract proverbs is presumed to have existed before the test was administered, although it was not specifically demonstrated until the examination; the same might be said for the physical, chemical, and metabolic aspects of the patient's clinical state. Thus, the clinical findings antedate the examination process.

For law, the conclusory findings—of guilt, liability, and so forth—do not "exist" before the actual process: It is the trial procedure itself that determines guilt or liability and the like. Thus, the findings in law are created by the actual resolution of the trial. By implication, then, courts create a certain kind of "reality" with their decisions (Gutheil and Mills, 1982; Mills and Gutheil, 1981). Whatever empiricism goes into the findings of law can then be selected (and, inevitably, distorted) according to suitability for inclusion in the trial process: Some evidence is inadmissible and hence it is excluded.

In certain situations, legal fact finders seem to believe that they can control external reality like the outcome of a piece of judicial decision making

(Gutheil and Mills, 1982). In other words, while judges can rule that a defendant is guilty, and while the ruling creates the guilt, a court will sometimes believe that its rulings can create external reality as well. An example of this occurred in the *Roe* case (*In the matter of guardianship of Richard Roe III*, 1981). The Supreme Judicial Court of Massachusetts ruled, without substantial evidence, that medications could "undermine the foundations of the personality" and that they were therefore "extraordinary treatment." The court seemed not to have tried to discover the effectiveness of ordinary medications as treatment, and just what effects on the personality they had.

In the main, there is no investigative tradition in law as clinicians know it. In a legal context, the term *research* refers not to prospective empirical study but to the search for past precedent. That clinicians rarely cite old literature bears this out: Clinicians recognize that new findings have forced old theories to be modified. (Of course, it remains fashionable to quote Osler and Freud, but beyond that modern formulations dominate.) To a certain extent, the law does the same thing: Novel conceptualizations can signal a pendulum swing in case law. But, law places great weight on precedent, that is, on what has already been done in the same or in very similar situations; experimental study is rare.

Replication and Follow-up. No matter how compelling it is, a single piece of empirical research is only suggestive until it has been replicated. If most of the results point in a particular direction, one acepts the conclusion as probable and notes contrary findings. In contrast, a single appellate court decision is binding on all courts below it, and it is likely to remain appreciably unchanged for years. This happens despite split decisions; there may be four dissenters, but a majority of five is enough to supply an absolute.

Rarely is the impact of any majority court determination rapidly assessed, and therein lies the rub. In psychiatry, as in other branches of medicine, if the treatment does not work, one is obliged to change course. Law evolves more slowly. With some exceptions, as when a decision is overruled at a higher appellate level, the law cannot readily shift gears. One of the basic principles of science is that of gathering follow-up data in order to evaluate the results of previous work, both for information and for professional accountability. While the law does not lack accountability for outcome, it makes little systematic use of measurement tools, and there is little or no tradition of empirical usage.

Final Thoughts

This chapter has examined some of the differences in the conceptual models of psychiatry and law in order to provide an underpinning for the discussions that follow. One reason why psychiatrists and lawyers reach different conclusions about such issues as civil commitment, the right to refuse treatment, and the duty to protect third parties is these conceptual differences.

However, differences in professional conclusions can also emanate from differences in values. The chapters that follow illustrate some of the conflicts in professional values.

Some of the cases in mental health law seem to validate the aphorism that hard cases make bad law. It is probably inevitable that, when law first considers a new and recondite topic, the first few decisions will be well wide of the mark of the ideal balance that successive reconsiderations can bring. Still, judging by the Supreme Court's language in *Youngberg* v. *Romeo* (1982), the courts are learning from the hard cases that certain decisions—about medical treatment, for example—merit review utilizing standards less rigid than those previously applied. To that extent, the courts appear to be making more than bad law in the hard cases. This leaning has an analogy in psychiatry, where it involves the so-called difficult patient. There, too, the initial learning may procede more slowly, but ultimately the therapist acquires a deeper understanding of the patient and the profession's techniques.

In the chapters that follow, the exposition of certain controversies in psychiatry and the law provides the necessary foundation for increased understanding across disciplines. It may also allow for a gradual ideologic integration.

References

Appelbaum, P. S. "The Supreme Court Looks at Psychiatry." *American Journal of Psychiatry*, 1984, *141*, 827–835.

Buchanan, A. "Medical Paternalism or Legal Imperialism: Not the Only Alternative for Handling *Saikewicz*-type cases." *American Journal of Law and Medicine*, 1979, *5*, 97–117.

Gutheil, T. G., and Appelbaum, P. S. "'Mind Control,' 'Synthetic Sanity,' 'Artificial Competence,' and Genuine Confusion: Legally Relevant Effects of Antipsychotic Medication." *Hofstra Law Review*, 1983, *12*, 77–120.

Gutheil, T. G., and Magraw, R. "Ambivalence, Alliance, and Advocacy: Misunderstood Dualities in Psychiatry and the Law." *Bulletin of the American Academy of Psychiatry and the Law*, 1984, *12*, 51–58.

Gutheil, T. G., and Mills, M. J. "Legal Conceptualizations, Legal Fictions, and the Manipulation of Reality: Conflict Between Models of Decision Making in Psychiatry and Law." *Bulletin of the American Academy of Psychiatry and the Law*, 1982, *10*, 17–27.

In the matter of guardianship of Richard Roe III. 421 N.E. 2d 40 (Mass. 1981.)

Mills, M. J., and Gutheil, T. G. "Guardianship and the Right to Refuse Treatment: A Critique of the *Roe* Case." *Bulletin of the American Academy of Psychiatry and the Law*, 1982, *9*, 239–246.

Mills, M. J., Yesavage, J. A., and Gutheil, T. G. "Continuing Case Law Development in the Right to Refuse Treatment." *American Journal of Psychiatry*, 1983, *140*, 715–719.

Mills v. *Rogers*, 457 U.S. 291, 102 S. Ct. 2442 (1982).

Rachlin, S. "One Right Too Many." *Bulletin of the American Academy of Psychiatry and the Law*, 1975, *3*, 99–102.

Rachlin, S. "Of the Shared Responsibility for Civil Commitment." *Psychiatric Quarterly*, 1982, *54*, 38–42.

Youngberg v. *Romeo*, 457 U.S. 307, 102 S. Ct. 2452 (1982).

Thomas G. Gutheil is director, Program in Psychiatry and the Law, Massachusetts Mental Health Center; associate professor of psychiatry, Harvard Medical School; and visiting lecturer, Harvard Law School.

Stephen Rachlin is chairman, Department of Psychiatry and Psychology, Nassau County Medical Center (East Meadow, New York); associate professor of clinical psychiatry, State University of New York at Stony Brook School of Medicine; and special professor of law and psychiatry, Hofstra University School of Law.

Mark J. Mills is chief, Psychiatry Service, West Los Angeles Veterans Administration Medical Center, Brentwood Division; director, Program in Psychiatry and Law, Neuropsychiatric Institute and Clinics; and associate professor, Department of Psychiatry and Biobehavioral Sciences, University of California at Los Angeles.

Because of the numbers of patients involved and because of obvious
past abuses, involuntary civil commitment has been the major
battleground between clinicians and libertarians.

Involuntary Civil Commitment: Legal Versus Clinical Paternalism

Robert D. Miller

Involuntary civil commitment cuts across nearly all the areas of legal involvement in psychiatric practice. In this chapter, I will concentrate on emerging trends in legal thinking and practice that have a direct bearing on the practice of commitment. I will use the term *legal* to include not only attorneys, judges, and legislators but also sociologists, historians, clinicians, and others who have influenced decision makers to restrict and regulate psychiatric practice.

Most discussions of commitment have concentrated on the direct effects of overt legal actions, such as law suits and legislation; I believe that it is equally important to examine both the theoretical bases for the positions expressed in legal actions and the attitudes that reinforce or resist them. Without addressing these underlying beliefs, it will be very difficult to balance clinical and legal rights.

Background

Western societies have always segregated deviant persons; Deutsch (1949), Foucault (1961), and Rothman (1971, 1980), among others, have documented this process in great detail. The handling of the mentally ill has been

S. Rachlin (Ed.). *Legal Encroachment on Psychiatric Practice.* New Directions for
Mental Health Services, no. 25. San Francisco: Jossey-Bass, March 1985.

marked by a series of reforms, each of which repudiated the principles and practices of its predecessors. When the concept of mental illness began to gain ascendency in the late eighteenth centrury, the mentally ill were formally differentiated from other deviants and placed in asylums under the control of medical superintendents, the forerunners of organized psychiatry.

There were many reasons for the absence of concern for the rights of these patients: There were no advocacy groups to protest, few statutes governed the process, and few judges were interested in the rights of mental patients. Reformers argued that removing patients from the influences that had caused their behaviors and providing discipline and humanitarian treatment in asylums would allow them to be cured (Foucault, 1961; Rothman, 1971).

As long as the patient populations remained small and highly selected, the cure rates reported hovered around 100 percent, and state after state built asylums (Deutsch, 1949; Rothman, 1971). However, as immigrants poured into the country cities became more crowded, asylums filled faster than they could be built, and conditions deteriorated drastically.

In the early twentieth century, reformers began to question the asylum concept and to criticize failures to cure patients; they argued for an individual, case-by-case approach. Their efforts led to the creation of outpatient clinics for the mentally ill. However, the asylums remained entrenched; censuses in public mental hospitals rose to a peak in excess of 550,000 in 1955 (Bachrach, 1976).

In the 1960s, the new psychotropic drugs made it possible for thousands of chronic patients to leave the hospitals. Prestigious clinicians argued that mental patients could best be treated in their own communities and called for the creation of a national network of community mental health centers. The civil liberties movement extended its efforts to mentally disordered criminals and finally to civilly committed patients.

Initially, the goals of clinicians and libertarians coincided to a large degree. The same uncritical enthusiasm that characterized previous reform movements infected the newest attempt to solve the problems of the mentally ill. Legislators were attracted by the prospect of financial savings from the closing of hospitals and by federal support for the mental health centers. However, it was not long before resistance developed. Staff of many early centers preferred to treat only the less severely ill patients. Chronic patients discharged from public hospitals did not voluntarily attend the few centers that were available, and their condition rapidly deteriorated. They lived miserably in psychiatric ghettoes, and many were often rehospitalized. Hospital staffs resisted efforts to close their facilities (Nelson and others, 1983), and community residents resisted efforts to relocate patients in their neighborhoods. The projected financial savings did not materialize, because hospital expenses continued to rise and because the costs of providing a full range of social services to patients in the community were far greater than predicted (Bachrach, 1976; Miller, 1982).

Litigation

Civil libertarians began using the law suit to speed up the process of deinstitutionalization (*Rouse* v. *Cameron,* 1966; *Wyatt* v. *Stickney,* 1971; *O'Connor* v. *Donaldson,* 1975; *Lake* v. *Cameron,* 1966; *Covington* v. *Harris,* 1966; *Lessard* v. *Schmidt,* 1972 to 1976; *Dixon* v. *Weinberger,* 1975; *Suzuki* v. *Quisenberry,* 1976). While clinicians at first supported the legal efforts (Stickney, 1974), it soon became obvious that many of the law suits were designed to abolish hospitals, rather than to improve conditions in them (Schwarz, 1974; Chodoff, 1976; McGarry, 1976; Wald and Friedman, 1978). Significant resistance to further court action began to develop. Clinicians resented the application of precedents set against substandard facilities to all facilities (*Rennie* v. *Klein,* 1979). State governments resisted courts' telling them how to spend money. Both sides dug in, and the original cooperation evaporated.

The reforms had produced some benefits about which both sides could agree. Many states upgraded their hospitals, and the number accredited by the Joint Commission on Accreditation of Hospitals rose significantly (Miller, 1984). Model community-based programs were established (Stein and Test, 1978), although not as rapidly as anticipated. But, while state hospital censuses fell, admissions rose, and outpatient facilities could (or would) not provide services for many discharged patients. Critics began to question the assumptions underlying deinstitutionalization, and federal and state support for aftercare began to decline. These problems accentuated the underlying philosophical differences between the clinicians and the libertarians.

Legal Reforms of Commitment

Criteria for Commitment. Basing their attacks on a small number of influential papers by outspoken critics of the medical model of psychiatric practice, libertarians put forth a number of arguments against the existing criteria for commitment: Even if mental illness exists—and there were claims that the concept was a subterfuge by which psychiatrists helped the state to exercise control over social deviants (Szasz, 1963; Shah, 1973–74)—clinicians cannot diagnose it reliably enough for legal purposes (Ennis and Litwack, 1974; Ziskin, 1975), and it should be a legally suspect classification and therefore subject to particular constitutional scrutiny ("Mental Illness," 1974). While these attacks did not result in the outright rejection of mental illness as a criterion for commitment, they did cast enough doubt on the *parens patriae* grounds for commitment to cause a significant shift in the police power justification. Although dangerousness to self or others was not yet definitively articulated on constitutional grounds, a series of court decisions (*O'Connor* v. *Donaldson,* 1975; *Lessard* v. *Schmidt,* 1972–1976; *Suzuki* v. *Quisenberry,* 1976) led to the establishment of dangerousness to self or to others as the major criterion for commitment, despite mounting evidence that clinicians cannot predict future danger with legally acceptable precision (Ennis and Litwack, 1974; Cocozza and Steadman, 1976). Some clinicians and judges responded by ignoring the requirements (Hiday, 1977) or by fudging the evidence for dangerousness (Wald and Friedman, 1978; Levinson and others, 1984). However, most accepted the changes and modified their recommendations accordingly (Gupta, 1971; Miller and others, 1983). This led to a dramatic change in the characteristics of inpatient populations; patients being admitted tended to have more severe illnesses and less treatable conditions (Sosowsky, 1978; Steadman and others, 1978; Levinson and others, 1984).

The Impact of Attorneys. Prior to the libertarian reforms, there were widespread claims that psychiatrists had far too much influence in the commitment process and that judges had abdicated their decision-making responsibilities (Cohen, 1966; Wexler and Scoville, 1971; Andalman and Chambers, 1974; Albers and others, 1976; Dix, 1976). While at one time this statement was accurate, the balance of power shifted significantly as soon as patient attorneys came onto the scene. A number of studies demonstrated that, whenever activist attorneys argued for release, most patients were in fact released (Wenger and Fletcher, 1969; Gupta, 1971; Miller and Fiddleman, 1983). A major reason for the shift in the balance of power was the absence of effective attorneys representing the state's position. Many states did not provide representation for the state's position, and those that did generally assigned the task to overburdened prosecutors, who took little interest in civil commitment (Miller and Fiddleman, 1981).

Despite characterizations of psychiatrists as anxious to continue their power over captive populations of helpless patients, most psychiatrists quickly relinquished their recommendations for commitment and yielded to the patient attorneys when faced with the prospect of serving as prosecutors. There were several reasons for this. Most psychiatrists felt that having to testify against their patients seriously compromised the therapeutic relationship (Amaya and Burlingame, 1981). Some felt that the time spent testifying could better be employed treating patients. Others did not relish the prospect of being cross-examined by attorneys (Gupta, 1971; Stone, 1979). Petitioners—most often family members—who were called to testify were reluctant to detail the patient's symptoms and behavior in court, so the formality of court proceedings acted to suppress the firsthand information that they could have supplied (Miller and others, 1983).

Plea Bargaining. The least-discussed aspect of criminalization of the mentally ill (Abrahamson, 1972; Stone, 1982) is the growing use of prehearing negotiations by adversarial attorneys. Such negotiations can result in excellent legal and clinical dispositions if the patient and the treating clinician are actively involved. Nevertheless, in practice attorneys and judges are making clinical decisions on the site and duration of treatment without input from patients or clinicians and often in direct opposition to the wishes of both (Miller and others, in press). In such cases, decisions are being made on arbitrary legal grounds without any consideration of clinical realities, such as the length of time required for certain treatments to become effective or the optimum site for treatment; such decisions may even be used coercively against clinicians ("Substantive Due Process," 1981).

Diversion into the Criminal Justice System. While there can be no doubt that these changes caused some patients to be released appropriately, many clinicians felt that the freedom to be psychotic experienced by the majority was a hollow victory (Rachlin, 1974). Many who would have been committed before the changes were made found their way into jails or forensic hospitals, where their liberty was at least as restricted as it had been in civil hospitals and where treatment was seldom available (Stelovich, 1979; Dickie, 1980; Sosowsky, 1980; Lamb and others, 1984). While strict libertarians, such as Szasz (1963), hailed this as a great step forward for liberty, and Monahan (1973) stated that we had not gone far enough in the adaptation of criminal justice procedures to commitment, one wonders whether we might not be regressing to the situation that prevailed when the mentally ill were not distinguished from the regular criminal population.

Patient Advocates. Legal involvement did not stop at the commitment hearing. Advocates mandated by patients' rights legislation proliferated within hospitals. While many provided useful services and were able to work collaboratively with clinical staff, others took the position that their job was to find abuses and to act as advocates for freedom, no matter what their clients wished. Trained as adversaries in the criminal justice model and cheered on by exhortations from the scholarly law journals, many did not realize that a number of patients actually wanted to be committed, even if they indicated a desire for release at the time of admission (Miller, 1980). And, despite a number of papers indicating that most involuntary patients were glad that they had been committed (Spensley and others, 1980; Toews and others, 1981), some advocates still refuse to accept that any patient can genuinely want to be committed and argue for release against the expressed wishes of their clients (Miller and others, 1983). A favored tactic has been the traveling hit squad of libertarian advocates who make the circuit of hospitals in an attempt to stir up business by suggesting grievances and law suits to patients who have not sought legal counsel or expressed dissatisfaction with their treatment (Brakel, 1981; Lamb, 1981). These so-called advocates are among the first to accuse psychiatrists of paternalism, without realizing that their single-minded pursuit of freedom from hospitalization and treatment is just as paternalistic as the psychiatrists' desire to provide patients with clinically indicated treatment.

The Right to Refuse Treatment. The next major offensive launched by the libertarians was a crusade aimed at recognition of the right of committed patients to refuse treatment. This problem, as it unfolded in Massachusetts, is discussed in Chapter Four. For the purposes of civil commitment, the importance of the right to refuse treatment lies in the fact that its implementation prevents effective treatment of many psychotic patients, thereby prolonging their hospitalizations—sometimes indefinitely—and leading to extended loss of liberty and additional suffering for patients, unnecessary costs for hospitals, and the transformation of clinicians into jailors (Rachlin, 1975; Perr, 1981). Without treatment, involuntary hospitalization becomes simple preventive detention (Dershowitz, 1973). In practice, relatively few patients refuse treatment for extended periods of time (Appelbaum and Gutheil, 1980; Perr, 1981), but the patients who do refuse treatment have a significantly negative effect on ward morale and on the treatment of other patients.

Treatment in the Least Restrictive Environment. The principle of treatment in the least restrictive environment (LRE) is not new; it was first articulated in connection with civil commitment in 1966 (*Lake* v. *Cameron,* 1966), based on District of Columbia statutes, and it was added to the required due process protections in several subsequent decisions (*Covington* v. *Harris,* 1966; *Lessard* v. *Schmidt,* 1972). Many critics of commitment automatically identified public hospitals with the most restrictive environment and used this identification to further their abolitionist views (Bachrach, 1980; Miller, 1982). Perr (1978) countered with a call for treatment in the most beneficial environment, but libertarians have not generally accepted this more balanced clinical view.

These early cases, and the statutory law that followed them, held only that patients must be treated in the least restrictive existing environment. They did not require that such environments should actually be available. Subsequently, there were attempts to ask courts to force states to create the required alternatives to hospitalization. Consent decrees agreeing to create community facilities have been signed in the District of Columbia (*Dixon* v. *Weinberger,* 1975), Massachusetts (*Brewster* v. *Dukakis,* 1977), Maine (*Wuori* v. *Zitnay,* 1978), and Missouri (*Caswell* v. *Secretary of Health and Human Services,* 1983). While some new facilities have been built (Okin, 1984), none of the jurisdictions has even come close to fulfilling its promises.

These suits were brought by paternalistic libertarians, who were convinced that they knew what was best for patients. Their efforts have spawned some resistance from patients who do not want to be deinstitutionalized and who have brought countersuits to block forced discharge (*Hildebrand* v. *Smith,* 1977; *In re Borgogna,* 1981; Peele and others, 1981). In defending against the suits, attorneys who had in the past argued vigorously that patients should have the right to make treatment decisions for themselves now argue that mental patients are not capable of deciding on treatment (Peele and others, 1981). It would appear that libertarians are just as prone as clinicians to decide that patients are competent only as long as they accept the "right" advice.

Liability for Release Decisions. There have been many attempts over the years to hold hospital clinicians liable for the behavior of patients whom they have discharged. Except in cases of obvious negligence, few of these suits were successful. Courts routinely held that clinicians could not be held liable for simple errors of judgment. More recently, however, following general trends toward consumerism (Wald and Friedman, 1978; Slovenko, 1981, and in particular the trend set by the *Tarasoff* v. *Board of Regents* (1976) decision in California (see Chapter Six for an extended discussion), many state courts have begun to expect clinicians to be able to predict future danger not only to identifiable victims (*Tarasoff; McIntosh* v. *Milano,* 1979) but also to random victims or to the patient himself. Even more recently, courts have begun to require clinicians to initiate commitment or to refuse release in cases in which they believe — or should believe — that the patient may harm himself or someone else (*Davis* v. *Lhim,* 1983; *Durflinger* v. *Artiles,* 1983; *Petersen* v. *Washington,* 1983). Since such cases arise only after some harm has already occurred, it is quite easy for a judge or a jury to decide that the clinician should have predicted it and taken steps to prevent it. As a result, the pressure to commit whenever any suspicion of danger arises is becoming overwhelming, causing unnecessary admissions and unnecessary extensions of hospitalization for many patients in order to protect potential victims — and clinicians. This trend will validate the criticisms of libertarians, who claim that psychiatrists are biased in favor of hospitalization and that they commit too many persons without sufficient reasons (Scheff, 1966).

Directions for the Future

It is clear from recent Supreme Court decisions (*Youngberg* v. *Romeo,* 1982; *Pennhurst State School and Hospital* v. *Halderman,* 1981) as well as from nondecisions (*Mills* v. *Rogers,* 1982; *Rennie* v. *Klein,* 1979) that the Court is getting out of the business of deciding mental health cases (Appelbaum, 1984) and even stating, albeit reluctantly, that clinical decisions can best be made by clinicians (*Parham* v. *J.L. and J.R.,* 1979; *Youngberg* v. *Romeo,* 1982). Lower federal courts can be expected to get the message, and the major channel by which libertarians have been able to impose their ideology on the commitment process will be significantly curtailed. Activist attorneys can already be heard gnashing their teeth (Perlin, 1981) and making plans to consolidate their gains (Paschal and Eichler, 1982; Lecklitner and Greenberg, 1983; Freddolino and Appelbaum, 1984). Courts are beginning to recognize that many of the proposed future reforms (particularly those involving the creation of effective community treatment programs) are extremely expensive, and state courts, in which most of this litigation will be heard, are becoming reluctant to make legislative decisions concerning the allocation of scarce resources. The current conservative trend in the country is another factor that may cause the interest of the judiciary in recognizing further rights for socially deviant persons to diminish.

Trends that are beginning to appear in various parts of the country exemplify this change: Families frustrated in their attempts to secure treatment for mentally ill relatives have begun to take a more active part in commitment hearings and to pressure legislatures to facilitate commitment (Simmons

20

and others, 1956; Freeman and Simmons, 1963; Greenley, 1972; Rachlin and others, 1975; Miller and others, 1983). The strict dangerousness criterion is coming under attack in many areas. The concept of gravely disabled, a throwback to the heyday of *parens patriae* commitments, is reappearing in legislative proposals, as legislators observe the consequences of limiting commitment to physically dangerous patients (Beis, 1983), and recent court decisions in cases involving pathological gambling (McGarry, 1983; Rachlin and others, 1984) and even shoplifting (*Jones* v. *United States,* 1983) suggest that dangerousness to property may be an acceptable criterion for commitment.

Thus, it may be that legal involvement in the process of commitment has already peaked. In the absence of pressure from the higher courts, practicing judges and legislatures are less likely to invade professional fields and to second-guess clinical judgment, and further inroads into clinical decision making may not occur in most states. The main area of concern now may well be professional liability for release decisions on the one hand and for malpractice in connection with the prescription of psychotropic medications on the other (*Clites* v. *Iowa,* 1982), areas in which the state has no financial liability and which are in line with the growing trends toward consumerism and antiprofessionalism.

References

Abrahamson, M. F. "The Criminalization of Mentally Disordered Behavior." *Hospital and Community Psychiatry,* 1972, *23,* 101–105.

Albers, D. A., Pasewark, R. A., and Meyer, P.A. "Involuntary Hospitalization and Psychiatric Testimony: The Doctrine of Immaculate Perception." *Capital University Law Review,* 1976, *6,* 11–33.

Amaya, M., and Burlingame, W. V. "Judicial Review of Psychiatric Admissions: The Clinical Impact on Child and Adolescent Inpatients." *Journal of the American Academy of Child Psychiatry,* 1981, *20,* 761–776.

Andalman, E., and Chambers, D. L. "Effective Counsel for Persons Facing Civil Commitment: A Survey, a Polemic, and a Proposal." *Mississippi Law Journal,* 1974, *45,* 43–91.

Appelbaum, P. S. "The Supreme Court Looks at Psychiatry." *American Journal of Psychiatry,* 1984, *141,* 827–835.

Appelbaum, P. S., and Gutheil, T. G. "Rotting with Their Rights On: Constitutional Theory and Clinical Reality in Drug Refusal by Psychiatric Patients." *American Journal of Psychiatry,* 1980, *137,* 340–346.

Bachrach, L. L. *Deinstitutionalization: An Analytical Review and Sociological Perspective.* DHEW Publication No. (ADM) 79-136. Washington, D.C.: U.S. Department of Health, Education, and Welfare, 1976.

Bachrach, L. L. "The Least Restrictive Environment Is Always the Best? Sociological and Semantic Implications." *Hospital and Community Psychiatry,* 1980, *31,* 97–103.

Beis, E. "State Involuntary Commitment Statutes." *Mental Disability Law Reporter,* 1983, *7,* 358–369.

Brakel, S. J. "Legal Aid in Mental Hospitals." *American Bar Foundation Research Journal,* 1981, *21,* 23–93.

Brewster v. *Dukakis,* Civil Action 76-4423-F (D. Mass. filed March 15, 1977); 45 CFR 84.4(b)5.

Caswell v. *Secretary of Health and Human Services,* No. 77-0488-CV-W-8 (W.D. Mo. Feb. 8, 1983.)

Chodoff, P. "The Case for Involuntary Hospitalization of the Mentally Ill." *American Journal of Psychiatry,* 1976, *133,* 496–501.

Clites v. *Iowa,* 322 N.W. 2d 917 (Iowa Ct. App. 1982).

Cocozza, J. J., and Steadman, H. J. "The Failure of Psychiatric Prediction of Dangerousness: Clear and Convincing Evidence." *Rutgers Law Review,* 1976, *29,* 1084–1101.

Cohen, F., "The Function of the Attorney and the Commitment of the Mentally Ill." *Texas Law Review,* 1966, *44,* 424–469.

Covington v. *Harris,* 419 F. 2d 617, 623 (D.C. Cir. 1966).

Davis v. *Lhim,* 124 Mich. App. 291, decided March 21, 1983.

Dershowitz, A. "Preventive Confinement: A Suggested Framework for Constitutional Analysis." *Texas Law Review,* 1973, *51,* 1277–1324.

Deutsch, A. *The Mentally Ill in America.* New York: Columbia University Press, 1949.

Dickie, W. "Incompetency and the Nondangerous Mentally Ill Client." *Criminal Law Bulletin,* 1980, *16,* 22–40.

Dix, G. E. "The Role of the Lawyer in Proceedings Under the Texas Mental Health Code." *Texas Bar Journal,* 1976, *39,* 982–990.

Dixon v. *Weinberger,* 405 F. Supp. 974 (D.D.C. 1975).

Durflinger v. *Artiles,* 673 P. 2d 86 (Kan. Sup. Ct. 1983).

Ennis, B. J., and Litwack, T. L. "Psychiatry and the Presumption of Expertise: Flipping Coins in the Courtroom." *California Law Review,* 1974, *62,* 693–752.

Foucault, M. *Madness and Civilization: A History of Insanity in the Age of Reason.* New York: Random House, 1961.

Freddolino, P. P., and Appelbaum, P. S. "Rights Protection and Advocacy: The Need to Do More with Less." *Hospital and Community Psychiatry,* 1984, *35,* 319–320.

Freeman, H. E., and Simmons, O. G. *The Mental Patient Comes Home.* New York: Wiley, 1963

Greenley, J. R. "The Psychiatric Patient's Family and Length of Hospitalization." *Journal of Health and Social Behavior,* 1972, *13,* 25–37.

Gupta, R. J. "New York's Mental Health Information Service: An Experiment in Due Process." *Rutgers Law Review,* 1971, *25,* 405–450.

Hiday, V. A. "Reformed Commitment Procedures: An Empirical Study in the Courtroom." *Law and Society Review,* 1977, *11,* 651–666.

Hildebrand v. *Smith,* Civil Action No. 77-0399 (E.D. Mich. filed Feb. 18, 1977).

In re Borgogna, 175 Cal. Rptr. 588 (Cal. Ct. App. 1981).

Jones v. *United States,* 103 S.Ct. 3043 (1983).

Lake v. *Cameron,* 364 F. 2d 657 (D.C. Cir. 1966).

Lamb, H. R. "Securing Patients' Rights—Responsibly." *Hospital and Community Psychiatry* 1981, *32,* 393–397.

Lamb, H. R., Schock, R., Chen, P. W., and Gross, B. "Psychiatric Needs in Local Jails: Emergency Issues." *American Journal of Psychiatry,* 1984, *141,* 774–777.

Lecklitner, G. L., and Greenberg, P. D. "Promoting the Rights of the Chronically Mentally Ill in the Community: A Report on the Patient Rights Policy Research Project." *Mental Disability Law Reporter,* 1983, *7,* 422–439.

Lessard v. *Schmidt,* 340 F. Supp. 1078 (E.D. Wisc. 1972); vacated and remanded on procedural grounds, 414 U.S. 473 (1973); judgment reinstated, 179 F. Supp. 1376 (1974); vacated and remanded on procedural grounds, 421 U.S. 957 (1975); judgment reinstated, 413 F. Supp. 1318 (1976).

Levinson, R. M., Briggs, R. P., and Ratner, C. H. "The Impact of a Change in Commitment Procedures on the Character of Involuntary Psychiatric Patients." *Journal of Forensic Sciences,* 1984, *29,* 566–573.

McGarry, A. L. "The Holy Legal War Against Psychiatry." *New England Journal of Medcine,* 1976, *294,* 318–320.

McGarry, A. L. "Pathological Gambling: A New Insanity Defense." *Bulletin of the American Academy of Psychiatry and the Law,* 1983, *11,* 301–308.

McIntosh v. *Milano,* 168 N.J. Super. 466, 403 A. 2d 500 (Law Div. 1979).

"Mental Illness: A Suspect Classification?" *Yale Law Journal,* 1974, *83,* 1237–1270.

Miller, R. D. "Voluntary 'Involuntary' Commitment—The Briar Patch Syndrome." *Bulletin of the American Academy of Psychiatry and the Law,* 1980, *8,* 305–312.

Miller, R. D. "The Least Restrictive Environment: Hidden Meanings and Agendas." *Community Mental Health Journal,* 1982, *18,* 46–55.

Miller, R. D. "Public Mental Hospital Work: Pros and Cons for Psychiatrists." *Hospital and Community Psychiatry,* 1984, *35,* 928–933.

Miller, R. D., and Fiddleman, P. B. "The Adversary System in Civil Commitment of the Mentally Ill: Does It Exist, and Does It Work?" *Journal of Psychiatry and Law,* 1981, *9,* 403–421.

Miller, R. D., and Fiddleman, P. B. "Changes in North Carolina Civil Commitment Statutes: The Impact of Attorneys." *Bulletin of the American Academy of Psychiatry and the Law,* 1983, *11,* 43–50.

Miller, R. D., Ionescu-Pioggia, R. M., and Fiddleman, P. B. "The Effect of Witnesses, Attorneys, and Judges upon Civil Commitment in North Carolina—A Prospective Study." *Journal of Forensic Sciences,* 1983, *28,* 829–838.

Miller, R. D., Ionescu-Pioggia, R. M., and Fiddleman, P. B. "The Use of Plea Bargaining in Civil Commitment." *International Journal of Law and Psychiatry,* in press.

Mills v. *Rogers,* 457 U.S. 291 (1982).

Monahan, J. "The Psychiatrization of Criminal Behavior: A Reply." *Hospital and Community Psychiatry,* 1973, *24,* 105–107.

Nelson, S. H., Vipond, J., Reese, K., and McKenna, K. "'Transfer Trauma' as a Legal Argument Against Closing a State Mental Hospital." *Hospital and Community Psychiatry,* 1983, *34,* 1160–1162.

O'Connor v. *Donaldson,* 422 U.S. 563, 95 S. Ct. 2486 (1975).

Okin, R. L. "*Brewster* v. *Dukakis:* Developing Community Services Through Use of a Consent Decree." *American Journal of Psychiatry,* 1984, *141,* 786–789.

Parham v. *J.L. and J.R.,* 99 S. Ct. 2493 (1979).

Paschal, N., and Eichler, A. "Rights Promotion in the 1980s." *Mental Disability Law Reporter,* 1982, *6,* 116–125.

Peele, R., English, M., and Redmond, A. C. "Is There a Right to Refuse Community Placement?" Paper presented at the annual meeting of the American Academy of Psychiatry and the Law, San Diego, October 16, 1981.

Pennhurst State School and Hospital v. *Halderman,* 451 U.S. 1 (1981).

Perlin, M. L. "An Invitation to the Dance: An Empirical Response to Chief Justice Warren Burger's 'Time-Consuming Procedural Minuets' Theory in *Parham* v. *J.R.*." *Bulletin of the American Academy of Psychiatry and the Law,* 1981, *9,* 149–164.

Perr, I. N. "The Most Beneficial Alternative: A Counterpoint to the Least Restrictive Alternative." *Bulletin of the American Academy of Psychiatry and Law,* 1978, *6* (4), iv–vii.

Perr, I. N. "Effect of the *Rennie* Decision on Private Hospitalization in New Jersey: Two Case Reports." *American Journal of Psychiatry,* 1981, *138,* 774–778.

Petersen v. *Washington,* 100 Wash. 2d 421, 671 P. 2d 230 (Wash. Sup. Ct., 1983).

Rachlin, S. "With Liberty and Psychosis for All." *Psychiatric Quarterly,* 1974, *48,* 410–420.

Rachlin, S. "One Right Too Many." *Bulletin of the American Academy of Psychiatry and the Law,* 1975, *3,* 99–102.

Rachlin, S., Halpern, A. L., and Portnow, S. L. "Abusing the Insanity Defense: The Criminal Gambler." Paper presented at the fifteenth annual meeting of the American Academy of Psychiatry and the Law, Nassau, The Bahamas, October 25–28, 1984.

Rachlin, S., Pam, A., and Milton, J. "Civil Liberties Versus Involuntary Hospitalization." *American Journal of Psychiatry*, 1975, *132*, 189-192.

Rennie v. *Klein*, 462 F. Supp. 1131 (D.N.J. 1979).

Rothman, D. J. *The Discovery of the Asylum: Social Order and Disorder in the New Republic.* Boston: Little, Brown, 1971.

Rothman, D. J. *Conscience and Convenience: The Asylum and Its Alternatives in Progressive America.* Boston: Little, Brown, 1980.

Rouse v. *Cameron*, 373 F. 2d 451 (D.C. Cir. 1966).

Scheff, T. S. *Being Mentally Ill: A Sociological Theory.* Chicago: Aldine, 1966.

Schwartz, L. H. "Litigating the Right to Treatment: *Wyatt* v. *Stickney.*" *Hospital and Community Psychiatry*, 1974, *25*, 460-463.

Shah, S. A. "Some Interactions of Law and Mental Health in the Handling of Social Deviance." *Catholic University Law Review*, 1973-74, *23*, 674-719.

Simmons, O. G., Davis, J. A., and Spencer, K. "Interpersonal Strains in Release from a Mental Hospital." *Social Problems*, 1956, *4*, 21-28.

Slovenko, R. "Malpractice in Psychiatry and Related Fields." *Journal of Psychiatry and Law*, 1981, *9*, 7-63.

Sosowsky, L. "Crime and Violence Among Mental Patients Reconsidered in View of the New Legal Relationship Between the State and the Mentally Ill." *American Journal of Psychiatry*, 1978, *135*, 33-42.

Sosowsky, L. "Explaining the Increased Arrest Rate Among Mental Patients: A Cautionary Note." *American Journal of Psychiatry*, 1980, *137*, 1602-1605.

Spensley, J., Edwards, D. W., and White, E. "Patient Satisfaction and Involuntary Treatment." *American Journal of Orthopsychiatry*, 1980, *50*, 725-727.

Steadman, H. J., Cocozza, J. J., and Melich, M. E. "Explaining the Increased Arrest Rate Among Mental Patients: The Changing Clientele of State Hospitals." *American Journal of Psychiatry*, 1978, *135*, 816-820.

Stein, L. I., and Test, M. A. "An Alternative to Mental Hospital Treatment." In L. I. Stein and M. A. Test (Eds.), *Alternatives to Mental Hospital Treatment.* New York: Plenum, 1978.

Stelovich, S. "From the Hospital to the Prison: A Step Forward in Deinstitutionalization?" *Hospital and Community Psychiatry*, 1979, *30*, 618-620.

Stickney, S. B. "Problems in Implementing the Right to Treatment in Alabama: The *Wyatt* v. *Stickney* Case." *Hospital and Community Psychiatry*, 1974, *25*, 453-460.

Stone, A. A. "The Myth of Advocacy." *Hospital and Community Psychiatry*, 1979, *30*, 819-822.

Stone, A. A. "Psychiatric Abuse and Legal Reform: Two Ways to Make a Bad Situation Worse." *International Journal of Law and Psychiatry*, 1982, *5*, 9-28.

"Substantive Due Process Limits on the Duration of Civil Commitment for the Treatment of Mental Illness." *Harvard Civil Rights–Civil Liberties Law Review*, 1981, *16*, 205-264.

Suzuki v. *Quisenberry*, 411 F. Supp. 1113 (D. Hawaii 1976).

Szasz, T. S. *Law, Liberty, and Psychiatry.* New York: Macmillan, 1963.

Tarasoff v. *Board of Regents of the University of California*, 17 Cal. 3d 425; 551 P. 2d 334, 131 Cal. Rptr. 14 (1976).

Toews, J., El-Guebaly, N., and Leckie, A. "Patients' Reactions to Their Commitment." *Canadian Journal of Psychiatry*, 1981, *26*, 251-254.

Wald, P. M., and Friedman, P. R. "The Politics of Mental Health Advocacy in the United States." *International Journal of Law and Psychiatry*, 1978, *1*, 137-152.

Wenger, D. L., and Fletcher, C. R. "The Effect of Legal Counsel on Admissions to a State Mental Hospital: A Confrontation of Professions." *Journal of Health and Social Behavior*, 1969, *10*, 66-72.

Wexler, D. B., and Scoville, S. E. "The Administration of Psychiatric Justice: Theory and Practice in Arizona." *Arizona Law Review*, 1971, *13*, 1-259.

Wuori v. *Zitnay,* Civil No. 75-80-5D (S.D. Me. 1978).
Wyatt v. *Stickney,* 325 F. Supp. 781 (M.D. Ala. 1971).
Youngberg v. *Romeo,* 457 U.S. 307 (1982).
Ziskin, J. *Coping With Psychiatric and Psychological Testimony.* (2nd ed.) Beverly Hills, Calif.: Law Psychology Press, 1975.

Robert D. Miller is director of forensic training, Mendota Mental Health Institute, Madison, Wisconsin, and clinical associate professor of psychiatry and lecturer in law, University of Wisconsin–Madison.

*Informed consent to medical treatment involves many factors,
including the patient's competence. What is competence? Who
decides? And, what information must the patient have in order
to give proper consent to medical treatment?*

Competence and Informed Consent

Robert L. Sadoff

Much has been written about informed consent in medical practice (Lidz and others, 1984; Cavanaugh, 1983; Weinstock and others, 1984; Meisel and others, 1977; and Stone, 1979). Lidz and others (1984) study research in the area; they present the decision-making process in psychiatry in great detail, and their work has been highly acclaimed. Cavanaugh (1983) contains several articles and research reports from a number of perspectives and for specialized patient populations. This chapter will focus primarily on the practical approach to decision making, particularly in psychiatric situations in which competence is involved. Do patients who agree to involuntary hospitalization have the competence to make such a decision? Do patients really understand the information that they receive from physicians about the need for particular types of treatment, including medication? Do patients have the competence to consent to treatment or to refuse particular types of treatment? This presentation will focus on the guidelines that have been established to aid practitioners in making difficult decisions about patients. Can the patient participate in the decision making?

Informed Consent

What is informed consent? How can it be distinguished from such other forms of consent as implied consent (wherein routine or standard medical testing is done on a voluntary patient), presumed consent (wherein procedures

S. Rachlin (Ed.). *Legal Encroachment on Psychiatric Practice.* New Directions for
Mental Health Services, no. 25. San Francisco: Jossey-Bass, March 1985.

are conducted on an unconscious patient unable to give consent but who presumably would have given it if competent and awake), or vicarious consent (given by the parent or guardian of an incompetent individual)?

Informed consent involves the giving of voluntary and competent consent by a patient who has received appropriate and reasonable information about the procedure or treatment offered, including morbidity rates, mortality rates, and alternative forms of treatment for the same or similar conditions. Lidz and others (1984) indicate that the multiple meanings of the words *informed consent* depend on the perspective of the interpreter. They note (p. 3) that the clinician views informed consent as a signed piece of paper "containing a description of the procedure written by a lawyer whom the clinician has never met." Legally, the concept is seen as a form of contract between the patient and the physician that establishes particular guidelines under which the treatment can proceed. Unless these particular guidelines are met, the attorney may see informed consent as a source of liability in a malpractice case against the physician.

What should the physician tell the patient about the procedure? How extensive should this information be? Should the information be written on the chart, or should it be provided as a standard form applicable to all treatment situations? There is no good answer to the question of how much information is reasonable and appropriate and how much should be written down. Both lawyers and physicians disagree on these questions. Some adhere to a broad view of informed consent, arguing that the physician should give as much information as possible in order for the patient to make a truly informed decision about his or her treatment. Others restrict the information to that which is absolutely necessary; they worry about burdening the patient with extraneous data that may confuse, rather than clarify, the issues. Most recommend against a standard form containing information about the various treatment modalities, because it will never be complete and because it can become a source of liability in the event of an untoward reaction or unexpected result. Most favor a fairly complete note in the patient's chart indicating than an individual discussion took place and describing the information that was presented to the patient in general terms.

From an ethical standpoint, Lidz and others (1984, p. 4) indicate that the broader, "more expansive ethical" reasoning can have two goals in informed consent: first, to promote individual autonomy and, second, to encourage rational decision making. These goals are particularly important in psychiatry, because both are geared toward the patient's growth; they do not foster the paternalistic authoritarianism so commonly seen in medical practice.

Models of Informed Consent

Lynn (1983, p. 31) presents a model of informed consent and decision making: "Valid consent is an assent by the patient or the patient's surrogate that (1) has occurred in the absence of undue coercion ('voluntariness'), (2) followed upon the provision of all relevant information concerning each available treatment choice ('information'), and (3) was made by a patient with adequate decision-making capacity ('competence')." Lidz and others (1984, p. 5) present a similar model in their empirical research on informed consent:

1. *Information:* What was disclosed, how, when, and by whom?
2. *Understanding:* What did the patient understand about the treatment? What were the important ways in which that understanding was developed?
3. *Competency:* If the patient did not understand, did he or she have the cognitive capacity to do so?
4. *Voluntariness:* Was the patient free to choose? Was he or she subject to coercion or undue influence?
5. *Decision:* What was the overall structure of the way in which decisions about treatment were made? What role did the formal disclosure play?

These two models are similar in the basic criteria required for informed consent. The consent must be voluntary. It must be made by a competent individual who understands the information presented and makes a rational decision about the treatment or procedures to be administered. A person may have the competence to understand the information given but he or she may fail to understand this information for reasons other than incompetence. The information may have been presented improperly or in a confused way. It is important for the patient to have the competence required to understand, but it is even more important for the patient actually to understand what is presented in order to make a voluntary and rational decision about treatment.

There are, of course, exceptions to informed consent about treatment, as in emergency situations. The rationale for such exceptions is that there is no time to make disclosure to the patient or to obtain consent without seriously jeopardizing the patient's well-being.

However, emergency doctrine for informed consent should be properly documented by the physician in charge and, wherever possible, by a respected colleague who shares in the decision making after personally reviewing the emergency.

The second exception involves incompetence. Some individuals are recognized as incompetent to consent to treatment. These individuals can be treated even without their consent. Whenever possible, a second opinion should be obtained about the individual's competence to refuse treatment or to consent to treatment. In some jurisdictions, the competence must be confirmed through court after a due process hearing that gives the patient a right to counsel and to cross-examine those who challenge the patient's competence.

Incompetence can be of two types, general or specific. General incompetence refers to a person who is actively psychotic, severely mentally retarded, intoxicated, unconscious, or senile. Specific incompetence refers to cases in which an individual is competent to make some decisions about himself or herself—for example, the handling of finances (see the next section)—but not the decision about treatment. Such specific incompetence can involve the patient's inability to make a decision, the patient's inability to make a rational choice, or the patient's inability to understand the information that the physician provides about the particular matter.

Perhaps the issue of informed consent was best summarized by Judge Cardozo in *Schloendorff* v. *Society of New York Hospital* (1914, pp. 129–130), "Every human being of adult years and sound mind has a right to determine what shall be done with his own body, and a surgeon who performs an operation without his patient's consent commits an assault for which he is liable for damages". The *Schloendorff* decision was upheld in *Canterbury* v. *Spence* (1972, p. 785) in which the court held: "In sum, the physician's duty to disclose is governed by the same legal principles applicable to others in comparable situations with modifications only to the extent that medical judgment enters the picture. We hold that the standard measuring performance of that duty, by physicians as by others, is conduct which is reasonable under the circumstances." These cases, then, establish that physicians have a duty to disclose information on which the patient can form a voluntary, rational, competent decision about treatment. The standard in the law is held to be a reasonable one, which physicians must define in each particular situation.

The standard of care is generally considered to be the reasonable manner in which the average physician would manage the particular patient under similar circumstances. The standard is, of necessity, open-ended in order to provide latitude both for the physician and for the patient. The guidelines cannot be rigid and overly specific, because one can never include everything in the information given, and no attempt should be made to formulate specific or rigid guidelines that cannot be met. Thus, in any case where there may be a question of competence or a question of whether the patient understands the information, it is important to have a respected colleague review the matter in order to establish a relative standard; otherwise, the decision may later be viewed as idiosyncratic if an unexpected reaction occurs.

Competence

Competence is a legal concept applicable to a number of civil situations as well as to a variety of criminal matters. Competence is determined legally by the court and functionally by psychiatrists. Of course, the final adjudication of competence belongs to the court following a comprehensive due process hearing. However, a person's competence to consent to treatment or to refuse treatment may need to be determined by physicians in a rather expeditious manner if the patient's well-being is at stake. There may be no time for a judicial hearing before treatment is administered. Thus, there exists the emergency discussed earlier and the need for vicarious consent by next of kin or legal guardians in the case of legally adjudicated incompetent individuals.

Generally, in both civil and criminal law, the term *competence* refers to an individual's cognitive ability to understand the nature and consequences of his or her actions and decisions. In criminal law, competence includes the capacity to give a competent voluntary confession or to understand the nature and consequences of one's legal situation with respect to standing trial, to pleading guilty, or to being sentenced. In civil matters, there are at least two dozen areas in which competence is significant. These areas include;

- Competence to manage one's own affairs (general competence)
- Competence to write a will (testamentary capacity)
- Competence to testify in court (testimonial capacity)
- Competence to enter into a contract
- Competence to get married
- Competence to own and run a business
- Competence to vote
- Competence to assume parental responsibilities

In general, competence involves the individual's ability to understand the nature and consequences of his or her actions or decisions in a particular situation in which he or she is involved.

Individuals can be incompetent for a number of reasons, including mental illness, mental retardation, and minority status (for example, if they are under the age of consent, as in cases of statutory rape). A person can also be declared incompetent if he or she is a spendthrift or easily influenced by the will of designing persons. The law is concerned about the conservation of capital, and it will uphold the incompetence of a person who tends to dissipate the family fortunes for the reasons just noted.

Historical Development. The concept of competence seems to have originated in English law of inheritance. The law of primogeniture dictates that the oldest son will inherit all his father's estate. If the oldest son was mentally ill, mentally retarded, a spendthrift, or otherwise unable to maintain or control the estate, the family needed a means of finding an exception to the law of primogeniture so that another son could inherit the estate. The method that was commonly used was that of demonology. In a certain sense, the demonologist was the antecedent of the modern day expert witness. Typically, the demonologist evaluated the family situation and declared that an incubus—the male demon—had visited the master's wife while he was away checking on his property. The demonologist's declaration typically held that the oldest son was not only not the issue of the lord and master of the realm but not even fully human, being half demon and half human. Thus, the oldest son was ineligible to inherit the estate, which would thus be passed on to the second son. Psychological understanding of mental illness and retardation has been refined, and the law now uses forensic psychiatrists and psychologists to evaluate individuals and given opinions about competence in specific situations.

Conflicts in Competence. A person may be competent in one situation and not in another. Determinations of competence are specific for each matter evaluated. Thus, an individual may be competent to write a will but not competent to manage his or her own affairs on a daily basis. In order to be competent to manage his or her own affairs, the individual must know the amount of money that he or she has, what form it is in, where is exists, and how it can be spent in a rational and reasonable manner. In order to prepare a will, the individual needs only to know the approximate amount of money in the estate and to whom he or she wants to leave it. There are instances in which an elderly person knows how much money he has and to whom he wishes to leave it, but he does not know in what particular form the estate exists or how to manage the money on a daily basis. Some matters require more cognitive ability or more competence than others do.

A particular case of such conflict was of importance in a recent criminal matter: A thirty-seven-year old woman living in an institution for the mentally retarded claimed that she had been raped by a fellow resident of the institution. The psychiatrist examining her for the prosecution declared that she was competent to testify in court, but because of her mental retardation, she was incompetent to give consent to sexual intercourse. The psychiatrist for the defendant found the opposite when he examined the complaining witness. He noted that she was unable to sit still during the one-hour examination, that she was not responsive to his questions, and that she often became violent and hallucinating. She did respond, however, that, if she wanted to have sex with her boyfriend, she would do so and that "no one was going to pay me $2 to have sex with a stranger." It appeared that she was able to distinguish between voluntary and involuntary or coercive sexual involvement but that she was not able to maintain a competent stance in order to testify under rigorous cross-examination.

Other conflicts of competence also occur, especially due to the multiple specific criteria in various forms of competence. Thus, it behooves the psychiatrist or psychologist examining for competence to be aware of the specific criteria for competence posed by the particular issue in question. Although competence refers in general to a person's ability to know the nature and consequences of his or her behavior or decisions, that ability always refers to a particular event, and the criteria vary with respect to each matter before the court.

Competence and Patients' Rights

Until recently, people who were committed involuntarily to state hospitals for psychiatric treatment were deemed incompetent as a result of their commitment. This condition continues in Utah, where commitment is tantamount to a declaration of incompetence. Restoration of competence requires a separate hearing following release from the hospital. Most jurisdictions at present separate involuntary commitment and competence. Individuals who are committed to hospitals are no longer automatically considered incompetent but must be evaluated specifically for competence to manage their affairs and to consent to treatment, and they are presumed to be competent unless they are declared to be incompetent. In the past, patients in mental hospitals were not allowed to vote or to enter into contracts because of their presumed incompetence. That is not now the case, since patients are allowed—and in many places encouraged—to vote, and they may also enter into contracts, purchase materials, or even get married while they are patients in the hospital.

The major concern with respect to patients' rights is the question of the individual's competence to consent to treatment or to refuse particular treatments when in the hospital. Some have argued that involuntarily committed patients should be deemed incompetent to decide on their treatment inasmuch as they could not decide on their place of their treatment—hospital or outpatient; thus, they cannot be presumed to be competent to decide on the type of treatment that they are to receive—medication or psychotherapy. Courts have indicated that that argument is specious, and in most jurisdictions involuntary commitment is not equated with incompetence. Thus, each patient within the hospital must be evaluated individually for competence with respect to any legal issue that might arise.

When assessing a particular individual for a specific matter, the psychiatrist evaluates the patient with respect to that matter, but, when the court declares a person incompetent, the incompetence is general for all civil legal issues. In some cases, however, the court may declare a specific or limited incompetence to the issue at hand, that is, to refuse medication or consent to treatment.

Case Examples

The examining forensic psychiatrist should make a comprehensive evaluation of any individual whom he or she examines for any form of competence. Particularly when the psychiatrist is asked by a physician or surgeon in liaison psychiatry to evaluate an individual's competence to consent to surgical procedures, the examining psychiatrist should be as comprehensive as possible. This means that he or she should conduct not only a thorough examination of the patient but that he or she should also obtain as much corroborating or negating information to the declarations of the examinee as possible. For example, the psychiatrist does not know how much money the person has or whether the statements that the person makes are true or false. The psychiatrist must then seek outside information from reliable sources in order to corroborate the information that the person has given.

In one particular case, an elderly woman was examined because she was refusing to have her right foot amputated although gangrene was obvious. She vehemently denied the surgeon access to her foot and implied that she would rather die than have her foot removed. She appeared to be mildly depressed but not significantly so. She was not directly suicidal, but she was clearly refusing to accept what had been termed a life-saving procedure. She was told that she would die if she did not have her foot removed. In this case, it was important to spend several hours with the patient in order to establish a good rapport and a trusting relationship. After ascertaining the degree of the woman's dependence on her husband and her need for gratification from him, it was determined that she was not psychotic and that she was not refusing on grounds of mental illness or impairment. She indicated that she had been observing the line of gangrene and that it had not ascended for the past three months. She was aware of the dangers, and she made her decision on a rational basis with full information from her surgeon. Finally, she indicated that she was not going to let herself die but that she would have the surgery if and when the line of gangrene began to ascend beyond its current position. She said that she was well taken care of by her husband, whom she had cared for during a ten-year illness. She had developed a balance of dependence with him, which she did not wish to disturb by the operative procedure at that time. She enjoyed the game she was playing with the surgeons and with her husband, but she indicated that she would be willing to relent at the proper time. She was, of course, declared competent to make the decision about her foot. Follow-up indicates that she had the procedure when the realized that the gangrene had ascended and that she was in danger of more serious consequences.

It has been observed rather cynically that patients are competent who agree to procedures recommended by the doctor and that patients are incompetent when they refuse. This oversimplified view is typified by a recent case, in which a young man was arrested for the brutal slaying of his homosexual roommate. While in prison he expressed remorse and confused ideation. He was able to obtain a razor blade while in the prison cell and cut off his penis in a fit of remorse. He was transferred immediately to the major university hospital, together with the severed penis, which had been placed in ice. Initially, he refused to have the penis reanastomosed to his body. The urologists, vascular surgeons, and special surgeons were all present and frustrated by his refusal. Many, who had been involved in a recent unsuccessful attempt to reanastomose another man's penis, were ready to leave when he refused. Others declared that he should have a psychiatric evaluation to determine whether he was competent to refuse the procedure. Psychiatric consultation revealed that the young man was not competent to refuse because of the gravity of the situation and because of his apparent confusion and depression. He was not schizophrenic, and he was not hallucinating at the time. Attempts were made to have a judge declare him incompetent so the surgery could proceed. All attempts were unsuccessful, and, during the period of negotiation with the judge by telephone, which the patient overheard, he agreed precipitously to have the surgeons reanastomose his penis. The question remains, Was this patient competent when he agreed to the surgery that everyone wanted to perform, or was he incompetent when he refused? No one questioned his competence when he agreed to the procedure, because it seemed to be the rational thing to do.

Another example bearing on competence and involuntary hospitalization is one that has been raised by a number of emergency room physicians and consulting psychiatrists. This example involves the concept that voluntary patients are preferable to involuntary ones and that voluntary patients usually do better in treatment. Most efforts in emergency assessments are aimed at having the patient agree to voluntary hospitalization when necessary, thus avoiding the involuntary procedures. If the severely psychotic, confused, delusional, and hallucinating patient agrees to hospitalization, there is little challenge to the patient's ability to make such a decision, and he or she is forthwith admitted voluntarily. If the patient disagrees and will not go voluntarily, the patient is then subject to an involuntary commitment if he or she meets the criteria in that jurisdiction. In that sense, the doctors declare that the patient is functionally incompetent to make the decision about where he or she should be treated and that the patient should be involuntarily hospitalized. Note that we are considering the same individual under the same circumstances: If the individual agrees to treatment, he or she is presumed to be competent to make the decision, but if the individual refuses treatment, he or she is presumed incompetent to decide and hospitalized against his or her will.

Conclusion

With the rise of mental health advocacy and patients' rights over the past two decades, we have witnessed major changes in professional attitudes toward patients' competence and informed consent. On the one hand, we no longer view involuntarily committed patients as being incompetent, and thus we tend to see most patients in the hospital as having the cognitive ability to make rational decisions for themselves, even if they are actively hallucinating or delusional. If a delusional system does not affect their ability to make decisions about treatment, they are presumed to be competent. For example, if a patient refuses medication because he is concerned about long-term harmful side effects, such as tardive dyskinesia, he is presumed competent to make the decision about refusal, and an alternate treatment may be provided. However, if the same patient declares that he is refusing medication because it, like the food he is refusing, has been poisoned by the staff, who are conspiring to kill him, he may be declared incompetent to make such a refusal, because his refusal is directly related to his delusional system.

Changes in law and adherence to patients' rights have caused attitudes toward patients to change in other ways. Patients are listened to, even though they may be psychotic, and even psychotic patients are allowed to participate in the decision making about their treatment. To the extent that patients are able in a rational and reasonable manner to make suggestions about treatment or to modify treatment plans, they should be heard, and their views should be implemented.

In summary, we can return to the guidelines on competence and informed consent recommended by Lidz and others (1984). In applying their general guidelines to specific situations, the examining psychiatrist should disclose the information that the patient needs to know in order to make a decision about his or her treatment. That information must be clearly understood by the patient, who is competent both to understand and to make a voluntary, noncoerced decision with respect to his or her treatment. This treatment is not confined to psychiatric treatment or medication; it includes any treatment in medicine, including surgical procedures, release of information, administration of medication, electroshock therapy, or various forms of psychotherapy. We must not neglect the will of the patient, no matter how ill he or she appears to be. Ethically, we are bound to adhere to these principles, because they promote individual autonomy and encourage rational decision making.

References

Canterbury v. *Spence,* 464 F.2d 772 (D.C. Cir. 1972).

Cavanaugh, J. L. (Ed.). "Informed Consent." *Behavioral Sciences and the Law,* 1983, *1* (4), (entire issue).

Lidz, C. W., Meisel, A., Zerubavel, E., Carter, M., Sestak, R. M., and Roth, L. H. *Informed Consent: A Study of Decision Making in Psychiatry.* New York: Guilford Press, 1984.

Lynn, J. "Informed Consent: An Overview." *Behavioral Sciences and the Law,* 1983, *1* (4), 29–45.

Meisel, A., Roth, L. H., and Lidz, C. W. "Toward a Model of the Legal Doctrine of Informed Consent." *American Journal of Psychiatry,* 1977, *134,* 285–289.

Schloendorff v. *Society of New York Hospital,* 211 N. Y. 125, 105 N. E. 92 (1914).

Stone, A. A. "Informed Consent: Special Problems for Psychiatry." *Hospital and Community Psychiatry,* 1979, *30,* 321–327.

Weinstock, R., Coplan, R. and Bagagri, A. "Competence to Give Informed Consent for Medical Procedures." *Bulletin of the American Academy of Psychiatry and the Law,* 1984, *12,* 117–125.

Robert L. Sadoff is clinical professor of psychiatry, University of Pennsylvania School of Medicine; director, Forensic Psychiatry Clinic and Center for Studies in Social Legal Psychiatry, University of Pennsylvania; and lecturer in law, Villanova University School of Law.

*The final version of an important right-to-refuse-treatment case leaves
paradox and puzzlement in its wake.*

Rogers v. Commissioner: Do Multiple "Wrongs" Make Patients' Rights?

Thomas G. Gutheil

The Boston State Hospital case concerning the right to refuse treatment
(known formally as *Rogers* v. *Commissioner of Department of Mental Health*) was
finally resolved on November 29, 1983, after crawling for eight years through
four different courts in five different versions — a numerical inconsistency gen-
erated by the case's having met one court twice along the way. Certain stages
of this odyssey, and certain conclusions of the last opinion rendered, make an
understanding of this case essential for anyone who wishes to grasp the complexity, inconsistency, and incongruity of this interface area between psychiatry and the law. This chapter proposes to convey such an understanding.

At one important juncture, the U.S. Supreme Court, having had the
case briefly in hand as *Mills* v. *Rogers* (1982), allowed the matter to slip through
its hands and regrettably avoided the opportunity to resolve the fundamental
clinical, constitutional, ethical, and moral questions raised by the right to
refuse treatment, the central question of this case. Instead, the high court
responded to the fact that, in the interval between the first *Rogers* decision in
1979 (*Rogers* v. *Okin*, 1979 — hereafter *Rogers* I), the highest court in
Massachusetts, the Supreme Judicial Court (SJC), had ruled on a state case,
In the matter of guardianship of Richard Roe, III (1981). That troubling, bizarre,

S. Rachlin (Ed.). *Legal Encroachment on Psychiatric Practice.* New Directions for
Mental Health Services, no. 25. San Francisco: Jossey-Bass, March 1985.

and extreme case, the wellspring of some of the most curious paradoxes in law and psychiatry (Gutheil, in press a), had addressed involuntary treatment of psychiatric outpatients. Readers interested in the *Roe* case can consult Gutheil (in press a), Mills and Gutheil (1982), Gutheil and Mills (1982), and Gutheil and Appelbaum (1983b). The U.S. Supreme Court sent *Rogers* back to the Appellate Court, which also had ruled on the case at an earlier stage, for consideration as to whether the intervening *Roe* case required rethinking of the Appellate Court's rulings. Out of several possible options, the Appellate Court chose to obtain an opinion from the Massachusetts SJC, that is, from the very court that had decided the *Roe* case in the interim. The Appellate Court did this by asking the SJC to respond to several questions. The questions proposed encompassed the central issues in the legal determination of the right to refuse treatment. The SJC debated the questions for nearly nine months, and the opinion that it finally delivered was a radical one in terms both of patients' rights and of the tension between patients' rights and patients' needs for care (Appelbaum and Gutheil, 1981; Rachlin, 1979).

The Judicial Context

In requiring that none other than a judge makes treatment decisions, the Massachusetts SJC runs counter in its thrust to important opinions from the U.S. Supreme Court and from courts in California, Washington, D.C., and New Jersey that presage a trend (spearheaded by the U.S. Supreme Court) toward nonintervention in the running of state institutions. Hints of this trend could be detected in two Supreme Court cases, *Parham* v. *J. R.* (1979) and *Youngberg* v. *Romeo* (1982). Those opinions generally found that—absent serious deviations (so-called substantial departures) from the generally accepted standards of medical care—certain forms of medical, clinical, nonjudicial review (modeled, say, as in New Jersey in *Rennie* v. *Klein* [1982] on the concepts of peer review or second opinions)—were adequate to serve the interests of due process while avoiding potentially dangerous and perhaps even unconscionable delays in the treatment process. The general viewpoint expressed by the courts was that physicians are in most respects ideally suited to weigh the risks and benefits of treatment for institutionalized inpatients. It is with this viewpoint that the SJC is most clearly in disagreement.

The Opinion

The essential core of the final opinion is as follows: A committed mental patient is competent and has the right to make treatment decisions until and unless that patient is adjudicated to be incompetent by a judge. If a patient is adjudicated to be incompetent, only a judge—not a family member, guardian, treating physician, or independent consulting physician—shall decide whether the incompetent patient would have consented to the administration of antipsychotic medications if he or she were competent. (This last concept is called *substituted judgment:* The judge substitutes his or her own judgment for that of the incompetent patient.) Moreover, the substituted judgment determination requires a full-fledged evidentiary hearing, with counsel for both sides, independent examiners and expert witnesses if requested, and so forth. If the judge finds that the patient would want treatment, the judge authorizes a treatment plan. No state interest justifies the use of antipsychotic drugs in a nonemergency situation without the patient's consent. Emergencies, as very narrowly defined by this court, constitute an exception to this rule.

As already noted, the opinion is organized around responses to the nine questions submitted to the SJC by the Appeals Court. These questions will here be addressed collectively for reasons of space.

The First Three Questions. The first three questions address the competence of involuntarily committed patients to make treatment decisions. The court begins by reminding readers that commitment is based on dangerousness and that "there is no requirement that a person be incompetent in order to be committed" (*Rogers* v. *Commissioner of Department of Mental Health* — hereinafter *Rogers* IV, p. 495). Significantly, the court seems to base its view on a point in the first *Rogers* decision put forth by Judge Tauro, who purported to find: "Although committed mental patients do suffer at least some impairment of their relationship to reality, most are able to appreciate the benefits, risks, and discomforts that may reasonably be expected from receiving psychotropic medication. This is particularly true for patients who have experienced such medication and therefore have some basis for assessing comparative advantages and disadvantages" (*Rogers* I, p. 1361).

Clearly, a court may rule that mental patients are competent until proven otherwise as a matter of law. But, in the original decision, this finding was a matter of law disguised as a matter of empirical fact. No reality-based evidence was adduced to support this dubious claim. Most empirical evidence (see, for example, Appelbaum and others, 1981) holds largely to the contrary; that is, almost half the patients sick enough to be admitted are likely to be incompetent. It could even be argued that, although commitment depends on criteria explicitly different from those for competence (thus, commitment and competence cannot be equated as a matter of law), making commitment the criterion may serve to select for the sickest patients, thus for those even more likely to be incompetent than the patient population in general. This conceptualization implicitly assumes that the committed inpatient is a basically competent individual who has some vague sort of disorder superimposed on an essentially rational core that is not materially affected by an impairment of the patient's relationship to reality. This basic misperception has been analyzed elsewhere (Gutheil and Mills, 1982).

In defense of its view that no less than a judge may make the decision concerning treatment, the SJC comments: "No other procedure is available for determining that a patient lacks the capacity to make treatment decisions"(*Rogers* IV, p. 497). This is sheer nonsense, betraying a disingenuous innocence of widespread judicial trends toward use of a variety of medical procedures in just these circumstances.

Questions Four and Five. The fourth and fifth questions address decision making about the treatment of incompetent mental patients with antipsychotic drugs. As already noted, the court opined that, absent an emergency, a judge must decide for the incompetent patient, using a substituted judgment. In an important footnote (*Rogers* IV, p. 501, note 15), the court makes this curious comment: "Even if the patient's choice will not achieve the restoration of the patient's health or will result in longer hospitalization, that choice must be respected. The patient has the right to be wrong in the choice of treatment."

"Rotting with Your Rights On". In a fashion characteristic of narrow visions of the issue of the right to refuse treatment, the court is here ignoring the latent problem of this view: For patients whom it is not safe to release, the clinician may be in the position of having to care for (that is, of having to keep in the hospital) a patient whom he or she cannot treat as medical ethics dictate. Such patients have been described as "rotting with their rights on" (Appelbaum and Gutheil, 1979). Thus, the patient's right to be wrong forces custodial care on the physician, together with attendant concerns, such as the rights of other patients to a therapeutic environment uncompromised by patients who occupy bed space and staff time without being meaningfully treated; problems with reimbursement for "untreated" patients; difficulties with utilization review; and so forth. This narrow view, which focuses only on the "plaintiff," not on the milieu, is, of course, an inherent scotoma of many legal decisions, particularly of the *Rogers* decision from its earliest version.

Least Restrictive Alternative. Even more strikingly, the court's explicit position that increased length of hospitalization is an acceptable cost of the right to make the wrong choice acquires parodoxical force when juxtaposed with the legally prominent doctrine of treating inpatients with the least restrictive alternative (Gutheil and others, 1983). Here again, the court appears cavalier in its lack of concern about the destructive impact of any increased length of stay on all patients in a ward.

The Making of Reality. The SJC further demonstrates its proclivity for creating reality by judicial fiat rather than by empirical observation (Gutheil and Mills, 1982) by noting that its own precedents have established the need for judicial approval before vicarious consent may take place to "proposed extraordinary medical treatment": "Since we have decided that treatment with antipsychotic drugs is such an extraordinary treatment [here the court cites *Roe*], we necessarily conclude that court approval is mandatory before forcible medication of an incompetent patient with those drugs in a nonemergency situation can take place" (*Rogers* IV, p. 501). Here again, the court, having decided that the most ordinary treatment is actually extraordinary, uses its own previous decisions based on this fallacy to demonstrate that its equally fallacious conclusion is thus mandatory.

Next, the court rejects the argument that the ideal persons to make

Next, the court rejects the argument that the ideal persons to make meaningful substituted judgments on behalf of patients are physicians or treatment staff. The court bases this rejection on its previous reasoning, citing from the controversial *Roe* decision: "No medical expertise is required [for making the substituted judgment decision], although medical advice and opinion is to be used for the same purposes and sought to the same extent that the incompetent individual would if he were competent" (*Rogers* IV, p. 502).

In one of the paradoxes to which the SJC is notoriously prone (Gutheil, in press a), the SJC appears to be ruling here without visualizing the actual clinical circumstances in which this matter might arise, putting patient and doctor in a Catch-22 dilemma. Since a committed patient, who may have triggered the commitment proceeding by refusing hospitalization, is now refusing medication, the patient must belong to a refusing/resisting subpopulation that tends to reject help. If medical input or advice must be invoked not according to need but only to the extent that the patient would seek it if competent, then the very patient who most needs intervention (that is, the committed patient) is also the most likely to have his or her refusal validated. Consequently, those most in need of treatment are the least likely to receive it.

The Adversary Assumption. The court reveals its inability to visualize a posture other than an adversary one by stating, "The fact that a patient has been institutionalized and declared incompetent brings into play the factor of the likelihood [sic] of conflicting interests [citation to *Roe*]. The doctors who are attempting to treat as well as to maintain order in the hospital have interests in conflict with those of their patients, who may wish to avoid medication" (*Rogers* IV, p. 503). As in many other adversarial conceptualizations, it does not appear that the court can envision that the doctor may want both to keep order and to respect patients' rights. The rights of other patients to a secure and therapeutic environment may be compromised merely because those other patients are not refusers, "plaintiffs," or the subjects of an assessment of competence. The adversary assumption of the legal process is unable to grasp that a synergy of goals, rather than a conflict, may prevail (Gutheil and Magraw, 1984).

The Court Hearings. The ruling in *Rogers* I, cumbersome and inefficient though it was, required only a single determination — incompetence — and a single action — appointment of a guardian. The guardian could then go to the hospital and participate in decisions without diverting staff time from patient care. A vastly greater investment of staff time is required under what the court advocates in *Rogers* IV: a full-fledged judicial evidentiary hearing involving "adequate notice of the proceedings, an opportunity to be heard in the trial court, and to pursue an appeal" (*Rogers* IV, p. 504). The costs in time and manpower are staggering: The procedure involves one judge, at least one doctor (the patient's, though other experts may be brought in), three lawyers (patient's, doctor's, and a guardian ad litem — a special investigator for the court), and stenographers, bailiffs, and hospital personnel as needed.

The court concludes that, after weighing the factors presented at the hearing, the judge, if finding that the patient "would want" treatment, should "authorize a treatment program which utilizes various specifically identified medications administered over a prolonged period of time" (*Rogers* IV at 507, quoting *Roe* at 1015).

The Court's Bias Toward Legal Sources for Scientific Information. The court enunciates six factors for the judge to consider (and to make the subjects of written opinions) in arriving at the substituted judgment decision; this matter has been critiqued elsewhere (Gutheil and Appelbaum, 1983b). What is particularly noteworthy and revealing in this list is the fourth factor, the probability of adverse side effects, elaborated on by footnote 21 (p. 506): "Dangerous side effects can occur even if the drugs are 'responsibly and competently administered with great care and consideration for the patient' [citation to law article by Brooks, 1980, p. 183]." The footnote refers the reader to a description of the adverse side effects of psychotropic medications. However, the citation is characteristically not to the pharmacologic literature but to the *Roe* case, in which the main sources of data were a notorious and biased lawyer's polemic (see later in this chapter); the article by Brooks (1980), a law professor; and a law review article from 1982. Typically, this court demonstrates its preference for legal sources, even when seeking scientific information; it eschews objective research and scientific evidence.

The court, hewing tightly to state law, then essentially rejects the various administrative concerns advanced by defendants, such as interference with hospital administration, increased length of stay, decreased availability of treatment, increased staff turnover, provocative nature of patient's illness, and various other adverse effects on doctors' ability to treat. The court then restates (p. 508) its conclusion from *Roe* that "commentators and courts have identified abuses of antipsychotic medication by those claiming to act in an incompetent's best interests." The court cites a number of cases as evidence for this point, two of which, curiously, relate only to mentally retarded individuals, with whom the use of these drugs is usually bad practice or controversial at least. Strikingly, all the "commentators" cited are legal sources.

The Data Base. This use of legal sources on clinical matters began with the previous case. As already noted, one of the most confounding aspects of the *Roe* decision (a major basis for *Rogers*) was the severe bias revealed by the selection of a distorted data base. For example, in discussing the effects of medication, the court spent eighty-two lines of the original advance sheet opinion in *Roe* quoting from the notorious legal polemic, "Limiting the Therapeutic Orgy" (Plotkin, 1977), which major legal scholars do not take seriously (Mills and Gutheil, 1982). In contrast, on this pharmacological question, a mere six lines were quoted from reputable psychopharmacological authors. The court then caps this legally slanted list of sources by citing out of context a single sentence from a clinical psychopharmacological article by Crane (1973), a sentence given here in its entirety: "Drugs are prescribed to solve all types of management problems" (*Rogers* IV, p. 509). No hint of the great variety of possible contexts in which this sentence could have appeared is given in the opinion.

The Court's Persisting Antitreatment Bias. A question that might be posed here is, Is the court truly antitreatment, or is it merely pro-choice, as it were? The data from the opinion itself seem to indicate the former. For example, in describing the obligation of the institution to protect third parties, the SJC once again commits a conceptual error, as it did in *Roe,* which telegraphs its fundamental antitreatment bias: "However, when public safety and security are a consideration in the decision to administer antipsychotic drugs over a patient's objection, the antipsychotic drugs function as chemical restraints, forcibily imposed upon an unwilling individual who, if competent, would refuse such treatment" (*Rogers* IV, p. 509 quoting *Roe,* p. 1018).

Not one but two paradoxical issues emerge here. First, the court appears blissfully unaware that it has made a prejudicial assumption: that the patient (whose only evidence of refusal is during the state of illness-caused incompetence) would, while competent, reject the medication. Thus, in a hypothetical case, in which it is impossible to know what the patient would have wanted if he or she had been competent, the court assumes in the absence of any evidence what it already knows: namely, that the patient would have rejected treatment.

But, the cream of the irony here lies in the view that anyone in his right mind would reject treatment: These medications treat incompetence (Gutheil and Appelbaum, 1983a). The central paradox of substituted judgment when applied to use of antipsychotics here detonates: It is never possible to determine clearly what medication a competent person would want, since this is tantamount to asking, If you were well, would you take medicine for your illness?

Questions Six and Seven. The sixth and seventh questions address emergencies or involuntary treatment by the principle of "police powers." After discussing the use of involuntary medications as "chemical restraints," the court concludes "that, only if a patient poses an imminent threat of harm to himself or others, and only if there is no less intrusive alternative to antipsychotic drugs, may the Commonwealth invoke its police powers without prior court approval to treat the patient by forcible injection of antipsychotic drugs over the patient's objection" (*Rogers* IV, pp. 510–511).

As noted earlier, the court seems to be blind to the inherent paradox of its interest here in less intrusive alternatives, when it has already preferred the more restrictive alternative of prolonged institutionalization to that of treatment and possible rapid recovery and discharge.

Even more significant and striking is footnote 26 (p. 510), which refers to the sentence just quoted: "The defendants suggest that certain patients, as a symptom of their illness, will periodically threaten violence. Predictable crises are not within the definition of emergency. . . . Therefore, in those cases the consent of the patient for medication with antipsychotic drugs must be obtained in advance, while the patient is competent and calm. If the patient has been declared incompetent, the periodic episodes of violence should be considered in formulating the substituted judgment treatment plan."

Under this definition, as I have noted elsewhere (Gutheil, in press b), it appears that California's recurring earthquakes could not be classified as emergencies, since they are disqualified by their predictability. I have suggested (Gutheil, in press a) that "the clinician and patient are caught in a 'rights window' whenever doubt is thus introduced as to the legitimacy of [emergency] interventions. . . . This hesitation then can itself cause violation of the rights of that patient and others by unnecessarily permitting even anticipated violence."

Questions Eight and Nine. The eighth and ninth questions address the relation of forcible medication to prevention of deterioration. The decision notes (p. 490) that the state may in rare circumstances override refusal of treatment to prevent "the immediate substantial and irreversible deterioration of a serious mental illness [citation to *Roe*]." While the words *immediate* and *substantial* have an operationally conceivable clinical meaning, the notion of *irreversible* captures the futility of the court's hindsight-based attempts to reason prospectively in yet another paradox: One cannot possibly tell whether deterioration will be irreversible or not unless the actual treatment is attempted in the service of reversing it; only when treatment fails over a prolonged period of time is the criterion fulfilled. Moreover, does this imply that, if later treatment reverses the illness, the intervention was retrospectively unconstitutional, because the allegation of irreversibility was found to be false? In actuality, the inclusion of this term serves merely to communicate the court's basic resistance to the notion of treatment in general and the narrowness of the loopholes through which it appears willing to permit appropriate medical treatment to slip.

Missing Elements

Some important elements are missing from the decision. None of the courts involved in this case has ever responsibly or appropriately addressed the question of what happens to the patient whose refusal is viewed as a competent and thus a supportable one. Many such patients, having been committed on the basis of dangerousness, simply remain dangerous if they do not receive medication. Thus, the patient who is substitutedly judged as someone who, if competent, would have wanted not to be on medication—a view that may well have resulted in the deterioration that led to the original hospitalization and commitment—and who would thus be viewed by the judge as appropriately refusing treatment—that patient is truly "rotting with his rights on" (Appelbaum and Gutheil, 1979), in that the ostensibly competent reasoning that got the patient into trouble in the first place is now invoked to keep him or her in trouble and stuck in the hospital for an indefinite period of time. Barring spontaneous recovery—a regrettably rare event—the path to treatment and recovery seems to have been closed judicially for such individuals.

Legal savants often advance the argument that courts at the level of the SJC are not seriously concerned with practical reality in the first place; they merely articulate the principles. As suggested elsewhere (Gutheil and

Appelbaum, 1983b), legal decisions of this sort become frameworks for the rationalization of decision making after the conclusion has already been reached on intuitive grounds; that is, having decided what to do, the judge then invokes the decision-making principles retrospectively to validate the predetermined outcome. If this suggestion is correct, the courts that make the actual decisions have the flexibility of much material to work with. But, in this fact lies the truly damning feature of the decision: namely, that it requires a full-fledged evidentiary hearing for each instance of presumably incompetent refusal. Since the burden of making adjustments in the program falls on the guardian or the court directly, a strict interpretation of the ruling, which, fortunately, is unlikely to prevail, would suggest that, for every alteration of medication, addition of ancillary treatment, or even dosage adjustment, an attempt must be made to obtain a reading on what the patient would have wanted concerning an increase in dosage were he or she competent. In addition, the following hypothetical scenario may bring the fundamental deficiencies of reasoning to the fore, in one of many paradoxical examples typical for this paradox-prone court: Assume that an incompetent patient who refuses medication is brought to the court, which draws evidence to lead it to rule that the patient would take medication if competent. On this basis, the patient is given involuntary medication and is quickly restored to competence. At the review, the now competent patient elects to refuse medication. The court honors this decision as competent, and medication is stopped. The patient deteriorates into an incompetent state, and the doctors bring the patient back to court.

The court must now choose between two previous conflicting but presumably equally valid decisions: the original one, in which it found as a question of fact that the patient would have wanted medication if competent, and the second decision, in which the patient voiced exactly the opposite intention when restored to competence. Since the first decision is presumably validated by the same care in fact-finding as the second, which is distinguished only by the more specific, in-court articulation of the patient's viewpoint, the court seems once again, as in the matter of substituted judgment, to give itself free reign to follow whatever it fancies about the proper outcome.

Conclusion

In a fundamentally dubious, probably biased, and paradox-generating manner, drawing on its own previous, equally dubious decisions, the Supreme Judicial Court of Massachusetts has taken a giant step backwards, which counters the trend of most enlightened jurisdictions in the United States, by imposing significantly restrictive procedural sanctions on the use of antipsychotic medications with unwilling inpatients. The court has attempted to achieve greater justice in decision making. It is likely that it has merely impeded good treatment in those limited situations where it may be available. Only time and direct empirical investigation will reveal the true cost of this decision.

References

Appelbaum, P. S., and Gutheil, T. G. "'Rotting With Their Rights On': Constitutional Theory and Clinical Reality in Drug Refusal by Psychiatric Patients." *Bulletin of the American Academy of Psychiatry and the Law,* 1979, *7,* 308–317.

Appelbaum, P. S., and Gutheil, T. G. "The Right to Refuse Treatment: The Real Issue Is Quality of Care." *Bulletin of the American Academy of Psychiatry and the Law,* 1981, *9,* 199–202.

Appelbaum, P. S., Mirkin, S., and Bateman, A. L. "Competency to Consent to Psychiatric Hospitalization: An Empirical Assessment." *American Journal of Psychiatry,* 1981, *138,* 1170–1176.

Brooks, A. "The Consitutional Right to Refuse Antipsychotic Medications." *Bulletin of the American Academy of Psychiatry and the Law,* 1980, *8,* 179–221.

Crane, G. E. "Clinical Psychopharmacology in its Twentieth Year." *Science,* 1973, *181,* 124–128.

Gutheil, T. G. "The Jurisprudence of Catch-22: Recent Paradoxes of Decision Making by the Massachusetts Supreme Judicial Court." *American Journal of Forensic Psychiatry,* in press a.

Gutheil, T. G. "*Rogers* v. *Commissioner of Department of Mental Health:* The Final Denouement of an Important Right-to-Refuse-Treatment Case." *American Journal of Psychiatry,* in press b.

Gutheil, T. G., and Appelbaum, P. S. "'Mind Control,' 'Synthetic Sanity,' 'Artificial Competence,' and Genuine Confusion: Legally Relevant Actions of Antipsychotic Medication." *Hofstra Law Review,* 1983a, *12,* 77–120.

Gutheil, T. G., and Appelbaum, P. S. "Substituted Judgment: Best Interests in Disguise?" *Hastings Center Report,* 1983b, *13,* 8–11.

Gutheil, T. G., Appelbaum, P. S., and Wexler, D. "The Inappropriateness of Least Restrictive Alternative Analysis for Involuntary Interventions with the Mentally Ill." *Journal of Law and Psychiatry,* 1983, *11,* 7–17.

Gutheil, T. G., and Magraw, R. "Ambivalence, Alliance, and Advocacy: Misunderstood Dualities in Psychiatry and the Law." *Bulletin of the American Academy of Psychiatry and the Law,* 1984, *12,* 51–58.

Gutheil, T. G., and Mills, M. J. "Legal Conceptualizations, Legal Fictions, and the Manipulation of Reality: Conflict Between Models of Decision Making in Psychiatry and the Law." *Bulletin of the American Academy of Psychiatry and Law,* 1982, *10,* 17–27.

In the matter of guardianship of Richard Roe, III, 421 N.E. 2d 40 (Mass. 1981).

Mills, M. J., and Gutheil, T. G. "Guardianship and the Right to Refuse Treatment: A Critique of the *Roe* Case." *Bulletin of the American Academy of Psychiatry and the Law,* 1982, *9,* 239–246.

Mills v. *Rogers,* 102 S. Ct. 2442 (1982) (Rogers III).

Parham v. *J. R.,* 442 U.S. 584, 99 S. Ct. 2493 (1979).

Plotkin, R. "Limiting the Therapeutic Orgy: Mental Patients' Right to Refuse Treatment." *Northwestern University Law Review,* 1977, *72,* 461–525.

Rachlin, S. "Civil Commitment, Parens Patriae, and the Right to Refuse Treatment." *American Journal of Forensic Psychiatry,* 1979, *1,* 174–189.

Rennie v. *Klein,* 102 S. Ct. 3506 (1982).

Rogers v. *Commissioner of Department of Mental Health,* 390 Mass. 489 (Nov. 29, 1983) (*Rogers* IV).

Rogers v. *Okin,* 478 F. Supp. 1343 (D. Mass. 1979) (*Rogers* I).

Rogers v. *Okin,* 634 F. 2d 650 (1st Cir. 1980) (*Rogers* II).

Youngberg v. *Romeo,* 102 S. Ct. 2452 (1982).

Thomas G. Gutheil is director, Program in Psychiatry and the Law, Massachusetts Mental Health Center; associate professor of psychiatry, Harvard Medical School; and visiting lecturer, Harvard Law School.

*Psychiatrists are increasingly vulnerable to lawsuits for
reasons unique to psychiatry, and for the peculiar irrationality
of many legal principles and procedures.*

Psychiatric Malpractice Issues

Irwin N. Perr

No physician can practice long in the United States without becoming acutely
aware of the rapidly and persistently expanding litigation system, which has
become a threat both to professional practice and to the rational provision of
medical services. On the one hand, we are told that the provision of medical
care in the United States has never been of higher quality; on the other, we are
confronted with increasing numbers of lawsuits claiming malpractice, failure
to adhere to reasonable medical standards, or failure to adhere to required
legal or administrative regulations. The claim, therefore, that the malpractice
system will raise the standard of care seems belied by the fact that improved
care has not been accompanied by a drop in litigation and by the fact that no
general relationship between litigation and overall individual physician quality has been demonstrated.

Much effort is now directed at educating physicians about their legal
vulnerabilities. The principles of law are carefully studied and expounded.
Many of the philosophical bases of American law have at least a superficial
rationality. Unfortunately, what happens in practice and in everyday life often
does not reflect the contents of laws, textbooks, or theory of the idealized
image of law so carefully nurtured by its propagandists. Juries act without
regard for legal rhyme or reason, and frequently the legal system itself,
whether judicial or administrative, blatantly violates any reasonable interpretation of law and therefore acts in what some might call a lawless fashion.

Those who study the actual cases have a difficult time ascertaining the

S. Rachlin (Ed.). *Legal Encroachment on Psychiatric Practice.* New Directions for
Mental Health Services, no. 25. San Francisco: Jossey-Bass, March 1985.

principles that guide them. Cases with almost identical facts have different conclusions. Here are a few examples: Lawyers spend a great deal of time selecting a jury. They know that the decision in a case will often be determined by the makeup of the jury—its attitudes and its prejudices. The jury selection system tends to seek out certain population elements, and the adversaries carefully consider the psychosocial biases of prospective jury members. While the jury system does minimize the power of government in criminal cases, the emotionally and political-social leanings of juries in civil cases are such that one might question whether fairness is possible in certain types of litigation (or, if fairness results, whether it occurs more by accident than by design). Unsophisticated juries with little technical or medical knowledge are asked to decide exquisite issues of relationships and causality where injury and damage have already occurred. If a healthy person walks down the street and is struck by a car, only the nature of the injury and its long-standing effect need to be determined. The issue of the relationship of the behavior to the injury is relatively simple. Yet, even under these mundane circumstances, distortion, confusion, and manipulation abound.

In cases involving medicine, the injured parties are generally those who have already experienced some type of deficit. They are the sick, who would not be under medical care if they had no health problem. Thus, any claim of injury must be parceled between the adverse effects of existing illness and the consequences of professional maloccurrence. Money changes hands only in the one case, not in the other.

Another aspect of the overall problem is the immense impact of the financial rewards available to all participants. The contingency fee system allows both for free litigation and for immense awards. In few areas of American life can any worker obtain so much money for relatively so little work as in this type of law. Since multimillion-dollar awards are not uncommon in such cases, the vision of riches shimmers before the practitioners of the forensic arts. They can obtain between 20 and 50 percent of the award. The temptation to profit is easy to mask with words expressing devotion to principle and equity.

Numerous parties benefit from the system—the lawyers on both sides, the insurers, the investigators, the paralegals, the typists, and a host of others. The entire legal machinery is put to work and given jobs, money, or power. It has been estimated that, in the professional malpractice system, 16¢ to 25¢ of every dollar in the system goes to the injured parties. The rest is distributed to the vast army that lives off the system ("Sue, Sue, Sue," 1975)—and this does not include the cost of the legal system itself, which is subsidized by government and therefore by taxpayers.

The legal system is put in the hands of lawyers, variously called attorneys, judges, legislators, and insurers. They all have a professional interest and ideology in common; elsewhere (Perr, 1976) I have called it the *JAILer complex,* by which I mean the judicial-attorney-insurer-legislative complex, and I meant *complex* as President Eisenhower did when he referred to the military-industrial complex, which has uncontrolled power over many areas of American life.

Although I could discuss many other aspects of the system in this chapter, I will limit the discussion here to the nature of the adversarial system by which problems are decided in our courts. In a criminal case, the image of two knights jousting in the cause of truth is both popular and dramatic; it is also sentimental. Significant criminal cases are subjected to exquisite scrutiny by the media, which acts in the United States as a check on gross abuse. A system of checks and balances exists, not by formal structure but by access to the public through the communications media. These characteristics of such a system are not usually present in the quiet courtrooms where issues of money and injury are decided.

Frequently, the champions of truth are assisted by so-called experts. The claimant needs an expert to state that the care provided was below that provided by the usual or average practitioner of the medical art involved, and the defendant requires an expert of his or her own to state exactly the opposite. Most often, then, each side provides a witness whose words contradict those uttered by the other's. If each side matches the other in number or in relative apparent quality or status, then the argument passes to the attorneys and the emotions of the decision maker. The expert only opens the door to these essential steps in the ritual. A peculiarity of the system is that there is no real control on the irrational—not even on a ridiculous or blatantly perjured stance taken by any of the participants. All that is needed is apparent sincerity and the power to communicate. Because the two sides are so often at odds, the jury is left to decide on the basis of its impression of who is the more honest. This explains why each attorney strives to disparage the integrity of the opposing expert witness.

The lawyers themselves reflect their awareness of the system when they seek professionals of high status and accomplishment who have not been in court before. Those who have testified are somehow considered to be tainted; obviously, there is more than a germ of truth in this posture. Tanay (1972) lamented that attorneys seek professional virgins (in the sense of never having been a witness in court before); he also pointed out that virgins are exalted in reputation but sadly deficient in performance.

Some professional experts or forensic scientists are people of great knowledge and integrity who have an interest in the legal process and in the ethical application of their science to that process. Others are knowledgeable people who sell their services for a fee; their main assets are their power of persuasion and their willingness to use that power as asked. Still others are people of meager talent who provide the ritual reports required for the multitude of lesser cases, such as those involving workmen's compensation and Social Security disability.

Once the attorney has introduced evidence to meet the technical requirements of the case, other factors determine the result. In an unpublished survey that I conducted a number of years ago, I asked chairpersons of neurology departments and heads of neurology residency training programs their opinion of the relation of injury to multiple sclerosis. About 95 percent said that there was no known correlation. In an actual case, there would be one representative reflecting the 95 percent view and one antagonistic spokesperson advocating the 5 percent view. In the courtroom setting, these two views would be regarded as equal. Confronted with a disabled and deteriorating individual, the jury may then be influenced to a decision for a plaintiff where the fate of that single pitiful claimant is matched against the government, a corporation, or an insurance company for an affluent citizen. My interest in this particular subject started when I read of a workmen's compensation case in which a garbageman had been struck in the head by a garbage can; there was no particular injury, and medical treatment was not required. Six months later, he developed initial symptoms of multiple sclerosis. The court ruled that there was a causal nexus.

Malpractice and the Nature of Psychiatry

The preceding statements are broad and have little to do with psychiatry. However, the issues just raised must be kept in mind, because they apply to all malpractice litigation. The terms *malpractice* and *professional negligence* refer to deficient professional care or to care that does not reach the standard shown by practitioners in the field. In the past, most claims of negligence were based on acts that a reasonable practitioner would not commit. Occasionally, the claim was based on the omission of an act that a prudent practitioner would have performed. As a result, there had been a patient injury directly related to the commission or the omission. The standard for acceptable practice of a medical specialty is that of accepted practitioners within the field. It does not need to be a majority practice, only one that is utilized by a reasonable number in the profession.

Even today, most lawsuits deal with positive acts or deeds, and these acts or deeds have generally occurred in hospital settings. Those having both the greatest adverse effect on the individual and the most clear-cut relationship have been surgical procedures.

Even if an effect is due to negligence, it is of negligible worth if it has not created significant or prolonged impairment. The loss for three months of the use of a limb due to a fracture has minimal compensatory value; the loss for a lifetime is clearly much more significant. The loss of a spleen is often an inconvenience; damage to the brain can be a catastrophe.

For these reasons, psychiatrists traditionally were not highly vulnerable to lawsuits. Psychiatrists see relatively few patients and thus their exposure is statistically limited. Much psychiatric practice has been that of psychotherapy or psychoanalysis, of which there are many variants. Inasmuch as there are many different standards, each of which a significant group within the profession finds acceptable, it is not likely that a given technique can be shown not to be within the realm of usual practice. Second, it is almost impossible to clarify either an injury or the relationship of a claimed injury to a specific treatment process. Third, the persons in treatment all have significant problems, which are often both longstanding and progressive, even with treatment. Thus, the rare lawsuits dealt with such issues as suicide in a hospital (usually won by the defense), an adverse reaction to electroshock therapy (fracture is not a reflection of negligence but a complication with a statistical likelihood, albeit low), inappropriate use of medication, missed diagnosis, failure to conform to procedures required by law, violations of privacy, and so forth.

Attorneys were not eager to sue psychiatrists. Even when suits were successful, verdicts would be relatively small. Many psychiatric patients have limited or nonexistent earning capacity, so that loss of future earnings was not easy to show. Expert witnesses who would testify to negligence were either not easy to find, or they were of such questionable character that they made poor witnesses. Like everything else, the cost of litigation has gone up, and most attorneys do not like to spend money on cases that they are likely to lose. (The vast increase in the number of attorneys with free time has had the opposite effect: a form of on-the-job training with limited cost.) Some psychiatric cases were clearly ones of general blatant abuse in a public setting and reflected the deficiencies of programs that had become unacceptable.

In 1975, the claims against psychiatrists were 2.25 percent per year; that is, about one in every forty-five psychiatrists would be sued each year (American Medical Association, 1975). To put it another way, a psychiatrist could be expected to be sued once every forty-five years, that is, once in a professional lifetime. With the recent rapid increase in suits, the proportion has now reached about 4 percent or once in twenty-five years—still much lower than the surgical rates of 20 to 50 percent, or the rates in some states for suits against all physicians, which range as high as 25 percent. In one state, in fact, neurosurgeons are sued on the average of once every two years.

The large increase in psychiatrists from 4,000 in 1940 to 30,000 in 1984 and the recent retraction in practice opportunities have stimulated some psychiatrists to enter forensic psychiatric practice, just as practitioners in other areas of medicine, particularly the underemployed and the underutilized, may be under some temptation to enter this arena. With better training and a sense of justice and social balance, others have felt a social obligation to participate in the process. Some do it for fun; some, because they like to talk and teach. Some do it for money; others, because of a sense that the knowledgeable are obligated to participate and not leave representation by default to others of lesser quality.

Much psychiatric care is provided in the context of governmental services. As consumer advocates and others examined the system, gross defects in public medicine became apparent, and lawsuits against practitioners within the system expanded accordingly, particularly since immunity provisions were gradually eliminated around the country.

Another reason for the increase of lawsuits has been the expansion of litigation beyond the bounds of a narrow malpractice or professional negligence concept. The causes of action have been multiplying rapidly. Each new cause of action that is recognized legally spurs litigation and claims for damages and awards. The loss of charitable or governmental immunity has already been mentioned. In recent years, there has been a rapid expansion in the use of the concept of lack of informed consent. Lack of consent, a complicated issue in its own right, creates special problems when the mentally ill are involved. Interestingly, lack of informed consent does not deal with the actuality of patient care or its quality. Therefore, unlike malpractice itself, which involves issues of professional standards and which therefore requires knowledgeable testimony about standards, the issue of lack of informed consent can in some jurisdictions be presented without the requirement of an expert. Most jurisdictions have required physician testimony as to what doctors tell patients, but increasingly the standard is that of what an average, reasonable patient would want to know, not of what doctors want to tell patients.

Such matters as failure to comply with laws and regulations in commitment, breach of confidentiality or privacy, assault and battery, outrageous conduct, duty to inform, abandonment, breach of warranty, defamation of character, and so forth have become better known to the more adequately educated attorneys, so that claims now refer to a multitude of professional sins.

A peculiar area is that of abuse of a professional relationship, particularly where the patient has been abused sexually or where the doctor and patient have become involved sexually while in a therapeutic relationship (Perr, 1975). The American Psychiatric Association (1984) has taken a strong position against abuse of the psychiatrist–patient relationship for sexual purposes. Such abuse is clearly unethical, and any psychiatrist who becomes involved sexually with a patient, whether for alleged therapeutic purposes or not, is vulnerable to suit. Should a social relationship with sexual implications arise, the psychiatrist should consider transfer of the treatment role to another therapist.

In psychiatry, claims have dealt with mistakes in diagnosis or improper treatment, drug reactions, suicide, failure to restrain, unlawful detention, improper sexual behavior, and breach of confidentiality. The first three have probably been the most common.

Peculiarities of Psychiatric Vulnerability

Until recently, the law was fairly reasonable in its application. Now a unique phenomenon has arisen. In medicine generally, most claims of negligent acts, as already noted, dealt with acts by the physician — misuse of surgery or treatment technique, adverse reaction to a diagnostic procedure, and so forth. When this frame of reference is applied to the practice of psychiatry, such thinking seems reasonable and appropriate.

Ordinarily, a bad outcome alone is not proof of medical negligence. Increasingly, physicians care for chronic diseases, which may or may not be alleviated but for which the ultimate prognosis is poor. Thus, arteriosclerosis, heart disease, renal incompetence, and cancers of various types are all likely to end in disability, even in death. Families and patients do not have unrealistic expectations. Physicians treating chronic disease do not fear legal consequences when illnesses progress, and organs slowly or rapidly lose their physiological capacities. A person has a coronary occlusion. Sometime, whether it be within weeks or within years, that person dies an acute cardiac death. Families accept death as a natural consequence of such a disease. There is no blame—at the patient, among the relatives, or at the physician.

In psychiatry, many of the adverse consequences do not result from direct physiological impairment. The problem often is not one of the physician's effect on pathophysiology. The result that is troublesome is a behavior, and the behavior is an act of the patient—assaultive acting out, suicidal efforts, drug ingestion, alcohol use. Anger is directed primarily at the patient and secondarily at the doctor. Sometimes, the prime target of frustration is the physician, who, the family feels, should have predicted, prevented, or controlled the behavior. This direction of emotion is often accompanied by guilt or blame among the family, and projection becomes an anxiety-alleviating device.

Psychiatry deals with behavior and its motivation. As such, psychiatrists have been considered to be wizards or magicians, Svengalis who can predict and control. These purported attributes have created expectations that cannot realistically be met. In recent years, the law has focused almost totally on the idea (or fantasy) of behavioral control in its dealings with the problem of involuntary hospitalization. According to current legal philosophy, hospitalization is not for the purpose of treating the sick. Its goal is to prevent misbehavior. If the behavior is recognizable as part of a discrete and treatable illness, then the goals of the law and of medicine coincide.

Where adverse behavior is not related to what physicians usually perceive as mental illness, then problems abound. This is particularly true for behavior that is socially determined or related to personality disorders or substance abuse. Here, admission is either inappropriate, or it does not have clear-cut criteria. There is no measurable endpoint in management. An alcoholic may be relieved of acute toxic symptoms within hours or days, but future behaviors will not be affected by hospitalization for the short-term effects.

Even if behavior before admission was "dangerous," dangerousness—particularly in the hospital setting—is not easy to measure. Dangerousness is only potential, just as a gasoline truck marked Danger has potential for harm. That harm rarely occurs, but when it does, the adverse consequences can be severe. Thus, when a patient engages in dangerous behavior on relaxation of hospital privileges or after discharge, the psychiatrist is accused of not having done something to prevent the danger, as if there were a specific means for doing so on an indefinite basis. Thus, psychiatrists find themselves accused of insufficient regard for the "dangerous" person, for whom some demand preventive detention.

Abuses of these concepts have been involved in many lawsuits. For example, a man had twenty-seven hospitalizations for alcoholism with paranoid features. After release from the hospital, he committed suicide within three weeks. The accusation was that he should not have been released. For another example, consider the mental patient who left a hospital where he had grounds privileges. He stole a car and had an accident in which another person was injured. That person sued the doctor and the hospital, as if the patient's behavior were predictable and controllable.

The focus of dangerousness in the public sector has spilled over onto the private sector. Social demands have a surface rationality, but in actual practice the psychiatrist cannot really deal with behavior except in the acute phases, where ongoing problems are recognized. Few recognize the statistical nature of the problem where actual adverse events are relatively uncommon when viewed in the perspective of the potential for such events. Courts have said that police, probation, and parole authorities cannot be held responsible for the behaviors of their charges. Prisons are not held responsible for the behavior of released criminals. Both reality and public policy recognize the unfairness of such demands. Yet, some would place such a burden on the mental health system. (The intricacies of the *Tarasoff*-derived cases are discussed in Chapter Six.)

Tardive Dyskinesia

Tardive dyskinesia is a mild to severe disorder consequent to the long-term use of certain medication. Its occurrence does not reflect negligence, because it frequently occurs without negligence. A number of regimens have been recommended to lessen the likelihood or to alleviate the symptoms of such a reaction. Therefore, from the standpoint of negligence law, its presence should generally not be a successful basis for a lawsuit.

One rational basis for a lawsuit is irrational use of the offending drugs. For example, it is likely that long-term use of phenothiazines or other tardive dyskinesia–related drugs for a condition not amenable to the medication would provide grounds for charges of negligence. While a number of steps have been advised—drug holidays and the use of certain medications, for example,—the criteria are not clear or specifically helpful.

Another basis for a lawsuit is lack of informed consent. Competent patients, or guardians or relatives of incompetent patients, need to be informed about the benefits and detriments of the proposed treatment. Paying attention to these public relations or communications aspects can deflect a later lawsuit. Since lawsuits in this area are relatively new, litigation is likely to increase over the next few years.

A number of years ago, lawsuits dealing with electroshock therapy flourished (Perr, 1980). Claims for damages were made particularly for bone injuries. Even if patients were worked up properly and treatment was administered in accord with accepted procedures, adverse sequelae occurred. Nevertheless, the defendants usually won as long as these steps had been followed. Similarly, informed consent was periodically an issue, but it is not one now, since permission slips usually specify the likely problems. The same will probably happen with tardive dyskinesia, unless a new and successful treatment for the dyskinesia develops, in which case new standards for treatment and recognition will evolve. Various psychiatric committee reports have discussed standards as guidelines for therapists—particularly for electroshock therapy and management of the risk of tardive dyskinesia. Similarly, the evolving drug treatments for schizophrenia and affective disorders have created new standards, with which practitioners should become familiar.

Suicide

Suicide or injury during a suicidal attempt is probably the greatest problem confronting psychiatrists. Suicide accounts for 14 to 25 percent of all litigation against psychiatrists, depending on the source utilized (Bellamy, 1975; Slawson, 1979). One cannot conceive of a psychiatrist practicing in the field of adult psychiatry without a constant concern that he or she will encounter a suicidal patient.

Every psychiatrist should be acutely attuned to the suicidal risk situation and to the clinical matters involved (Perr, 1965, 1974, 1978, 1979; Rachlin, 1984). The demographics of suicide provide statistical information that is only relatively helpful in determining risk. This chapter is not the place for a detailed discussion of suicide data, relation to diagnosis, age, sex, race, cultural background, social supports, and so forth, particularly in view of the very voluminous literature on suicide. The focus here is on the litigation risk and on what should be reasonable law.

At least 30,000 die by suicide a year. (The true number is probably more than 50,000.) Several hundred such deaths a year occur in hospitals—both general and psychiatric. A small number of the hospital suicides—one estimate is one third—result in litigation. A high percentage of people who do commit suicide have seen a mental health professional within the prior year.

Suicide occurs to two psychiatric populations, outpatients and inpatients. The legal issues are somewhat different in the two cases. The only claim that is usually made concerning outpatients is either that the patient should have been hospitalized and the suicide thus prevented or that the patient should not have been released if he or she had been hospitalized. Such claims are rarely successful for a number of reasons. One is the general recognition of the problem of predictability and the need for clinical judgment. Depression in one form or another, whether in association with affective disorder or another psychiatric symptom complex, is extremely common. Depressive features may be prominent in 25 percent to 50 percent of the patients seen. Usually, hospitalization is considered for psychotic depressions, which are definable and measurable. The medical focus is the treatment of the affective disorder, and the degree of symptomatology, particularly in an endogenous depression, can be measured by a reasonably accepted set of standards. Patient management is complicated by many conditions, including chronic depression, alcohol and drug problems, and chaotic disorders, such as schizophrenia, where the proportion of suicides to the total number of patients is low, but suicide does occur. A "lesser" illness, such as chronic alcoholism, apparently has a much higher suicide rate.

Many people are chronically depressed and exhibit a dysthymic orientation. There is no measurable endpoint for admission or discharge. Hospital treatment is not particularly efficacious. Suicidality may be affected by situational stress and other factors, such as physical illness, which are not predictable or controllable.

Some groups seem to have a relatively low suicide rate. As mentioned, many feel that depressive neurotics have a low rate compared to those with major affective disorders. Personality disorders, particularly passive-aggressive and antisocial personalities, can be accompanied by suicidality, but suicide is not predictable. Suicide by people with personality disorders, frequently seen in jails, reflects this unpredictability.

Sometimes, the law has simplistically required for an individual to have attempted or threatened suicide as the condition for involuntary admission. Yet, this is not a good clinical criterion. Adolescents and young adults frequently make threats and gestures, but they show little intent to die, their efforts are rarely lethal, their efforts have a manipulative element, or they arrange for rescue. Hysterics and emotionally labile people in particular fit these categories. In one community, 0.4 percent of the population attempted suicide in one year by drug ingestion (O'Brien, 1977).

Clinical evaluation requires a global clinical judgment. Where that judgment has been made but where the records do not describe the data on which the judgment was based, the defendant psychiatrist is placed in a more difficult position than would have been the case if the reporting had been adequate. In hospital practice, the situation is somewhat different. An attempt to measure the degree of depression should be part of the mental status examination of depressed patients.

The most crucial type of case is the one in which the patient has been recognized as being suicidal as a result of the correlation of historical data with the mental status review. Generally, at this point, no laboratory procedures, whether psychological testing or neuroendocrine studies, provide reliable guidelines. Where suicidality is considered a current risk, some hospital procedure is necessary. The procedures to be used, whether they be periodic observation, close observation, one-on-one supervision, seclusion, or restriction to the ward, should be spelled out within the hospital. If nothing is done, the usual claim is that the psychiatrist should have known of an imminent suicidal risk and did not act. While rare, factual circumstances may occasionally support a claim of ignorance of a risk which should have been recognized.

Because of the problems in individual assessment, hospitals should consider general means for decreasing the opportunities for suicide. The most important means is the unbreakable or screened window. Jumping constituted 28 percent of the suicides in a survey that I conducted. Thus, it may be helpful to limit the opportunities for jumping. The most common method was hanging—41 percent. This is extremely difficult to control, because clothes, sheets, and places from which to hang are readily available. Other modes are overdosage, cutting, and jumping in front of a vehicle. Since hospitals are not prisons, overdosage is difficult to control.

I have reviewed thirty-four cases for attorneys in suicide litigation—whether for completed suicide or for injury related to a purported suicide attempt. Of the first thirty-two suicides, 40.6 percent involved hanging, 28.1 percent jumping or falling, 9.4 percent jumping in front of a vehicle, 9.4 percent exposure, 6.3 percent wristcutting, 3.1 percent overdose, and 3.1 percent shooting. The last two were outpatient occurrences. Thirty-one percent occurred in a general hospital psychiatric unit, 25 percent in a government psychiatric hospital, 12.5 percent in a general hospital nonpsychiatric unit, and 12.5 percent in a private psychiatric hospital; 15.6 percent were not hospitalized, and 3.1 percent occurred in prison. The psychiatric disorders covered the spectrum of conditions seen by psychiatrists. The age distribution was striking and did not conform to clinical expectations. None of the cases involved an individual over age sixty-five; 10.9 percent were over age forty-five, and 43.8 percent were in the fifteen- to twenty-four-year-old group. Among those in the last group, borderline personality and bipolar disorder were frequent. The borderline group is particularly difficult because of the symptoms are amorphous, there are few accepted or viable treatment programs, and the problems themselves are chronic.

The matter of adequate records has already been mentioned. If one can show what was done and why, one is more likely to provide justification for the procedures used. Since most claims are based on alleged omissions by the therapist, rather than on commission of negligent acts, adequate records are particularly helpful. As it is, trying to justify a negative act is difficult enough, like proving that one was not a Communist.

A second area of malpractice claim involves the allegation that change in precautions or patient status was not justified. A significant number of these cases have involved suicide after such a change, such as the granting of off-ward privileges, the granting of grounds privileges, or discharge. When suicidal precautions are discontinued or significant changes in the degree of supervision are made, a note should be made describing the basis for the change.

Some experts for plaintiffs claim that, because the patient had improved, the patient thus had a higher energy level and was therefore at increased risk for suicide. This type of thinking, to my mind, is not acceptable. The only criterion for the psychiatrist is clinical improvement in the patient, and using any other measuring stick would create an impossible situation, or to put it more accurately, there would be no measuring stick at all.

In my opinion, suicide should be a rare case for legitimate litigation. However, at least 10 percent of the suicides in my series represented situations in which the care that had been given was below the accepted professional standards.

Conclusion

Litigation poses an increasing threat to psychiatric practice. While some cases represent acceptable claims within the framework of traditional law, others reflect a chaotic, inconsistent, and unreasonable attempt to place blame on psychiatrists for the actions of their patients. Knowledge of potential problems can aid in risk management, but in the long run, only a reorientation of the law and a searching inquiry into the evidentiary and damage systems will provide any meaningful relief.

References

American Medical Association. *Malpractice in Focus.* Chicago: American Medical Association, 1975.

American Psychiatric Association. *Principles of Medical Ethics with Annotations Especially Applicable to Psychiatry.* Washington, D.C.: American Psychiatric Association, 1984.

Bellamy, W. A. "Psychiatric Malpractice." In D. X. Freedman and J. E. Dyrud (Eds.), *American Handbook of Psychiatry.* Vol. 5. New York: Basic Books, 1975.

O'Brien, P. "Increase in Suicide Attempts by Drug Ingestion: The Boston Experience, 1964-1974." *Archives of General Psychiatry,* 1977, *34,* 1165-1169.

Perr, I. N. "Liability of Hospital and Psychiatrist in Suicide." *American Journal of Psychiatry,* 1965, *122,* 631-638.

Perr, I. N. "Suicide and Civil Litigation." *Journal of Forensic Sciences,* 1974, *19,* 261-266.

Perr, I. N. "Legal Aspects of Sexual Therapies." *Journal of Legal Medicine,* 1975, *3* (1), 33-38.

Perr, I. N. "The Great JAILer Conspiracy—Malpractice, Torts, and the Middle Class." *Journal of Legal Medicine,* 1976, *4* (3), 16-19.

Perr. I. N. "Legal Aspects of Suicide." *Legal Aspects of Medical Practice,* 1978, *6* (1), 49-55.

Perr, I. N. "Legal Aspects of Suicide." In L. D. Hankoff and B. Einsidler (Eds.), *Suicide: Theory and Clinical Aspects.* Littleton, Mass.: PSG Publishing, 1979.

Perr, I. N. "Liability and Electroshock Therapy." *Journal of Forensic Sciences,* 1980, *25,* 508-513.

Rachlin, S. "Double Jeopardy: Suicide and Malpractice." *General Hospital Psychiatry,* 1984, *6,* 302-307.

Slawson, P. F. "Psychiatric Malpractice: The California Experience." *American Journal of Psychiatry,* 1979, *136,* 650-654.

"Sue! Sue! Sue!" *Forbes,* September 1, 1975, p. 63.

Tanay, E. "Forensic Psychiatry in the Legal Defense of Murder." *Journal of Forensic Sciences,* 1972, *17,* 15-24.

Irwin N. Perr is professor of psychiatry, Rutgers Medical School, University of Medicine and Dentistry of New Jersey, and adjunct professor of law, Rutgers Law School–Newark.

*The psychotherapeutic duty to protect third parties from a patient's
violent acts is a reasonable societal obligation, so a similar duty
should be recognized for all who routinely have special access to
information about violence.*

Expanding the Duties to Protect Third Parties from Violent Acts

Mark J. Mills

No area of litigation involving psychotherapists appears as active as suits arising from the *Tarasoff* duty. More than twenty cases have been reported since the start of 1980 (Mills, 1984a), and even more recent cases can be added (*Hamilton v. Reynolds*, 1983; *Whalen v. Nevada*, 1984; *Clark v. New York*, 1984). The *Tarasoff* case, now well known to nearly all psychotherapists (Roth, 1977), has been the source of considerable controversy (Stone, 1976). Givelber and others (1984) have demonstrated convincingly that most psychotherapists believe that warning the known, intended victim fully satisfies the *Tarasoff* obligations (Runch, 1984). However, Kroll and Mackenzie (1983), Appelbaum (1984), Wettstein (1984), and Mills (1984a) have stressed that this is not the case. The duties emanating from *Tarasoff* and its legal progeny (Mills, 1984b) require psychotherapists to protect, not necessarily to warn, the intended victim (but see LeBlang, 1982).

Using *Tarasoff* Clinically

Presumably, providing protection may entail a good deal more than warning. More important, by structuring the *Tarasoff* duty as a duty to protect, the courts have provided psychotherapists with a rule that encourages clinical solutions to the problem of caring for intended victims. Rather than being

S. Rachlin (Ed.). *Legal Encroachment on Psychiatric Practice.* New Directions for
Mental Health Services, no. 25. San Francisco: Jossey-Bass, March 1985.

obligated to warn, the therapist faced with a threatening patient has a wide array of options. First, of course, he or she needs to enquire specifically about the patient's verbalization; for example, "Did I hear you correctly, Mr. Smith, that you sometimes feel like hurting your wife?" If such routine therapeutic investigation reveals that the patient is actually harboring thoughts of hurting another, then the task becomes one of understanding the clinical import of such thoughts (Mills, 1984a). Fantasies of hurting another mean one thing if the patient has no history of previous violent behavior and possesses a well-developed superego and another if the patient has been repetitively assaultive.

Assuming for the sake of illustration that one is facing a clinical situation akin to the latter, the *Tarasoff* doctrine encourages clinical flexibility. If the patient is not presently psychotic, one can act to protect the intended victim by working clinically to keep the patient nonpsychotic. Such work might include encouraging the patient to continue taking neuroleptic medication (Berger, 1978). Alternatively, if the patient demonstrates psychotic features, the therapist can act to protect the intended victim by increasing the dosage of medication, changing the medication, hospitalizing the patient, civilly committing the patient, or combining some of these alternatives.

This list of clinical alternatives is far from comprehensive. Often, the clinician will have the time to obtain one or several relevant consultations. With the patient who is only violent when psychotic, and who is decompensating, an initial consultation might be psychotherapeutic or pharmacological. However, if the patient's psychosis worsens, one might arrange a consultation with an expert in the clinical assessment and management of violent behavior. Finally, if the patient's threats escalate, one might choose to consult a forensic psychiatrist, an attorney, or both in order to consider the most clinically efficacious manner of discharging the *Tarasoff* duty to protect the intended victim.

Warning. A bill was passed by the California state legislature and vetoed by the governor that would provide for statutory immunity from civil suit in cases where the psychotherapist warns a victim but injury or death occurs nonetheless. Both the California Psychological Association and the California Psychiatric Association have worked to support the legislation, apparently in the belief that their members would appreciate the certainty of knowing that they could guard against liability by warning. If the bill had passed, one could have anticipated that therapists would have warned whenever there was reasonable doubt about a patient's propensity for violence. That is, one can imagine that the use of warning to discharge the *Tarasoff* duty will increase. This aspect of the proposed legislation is unfortunate. Although *Tarasoff* II (1976) is sometimes criticized for having further extended the duty imposed by *Tarasoff* I (1974), reshaping the duty to warn as the duty to protect has meant that the duty can generally be discharged without having to warn.

This fact has had a number of advantages for patients and therapists. First, it has meant that the patient's confidences have been protected (Slovenko, 1975). Second, it has meant that therapists have been sued less frequently than in the past for violating patients' confidences. Third, it has minimized the consequences of false predictions of violence: It is one thing to ask a patient to increase his or her medications and later decide that the increase was unwarranted and another to involve a third party, who in some cases will be always wary of the patient thereafter. Fourth and most important, the clinical interventions practiced to protect third parties can occur where the identity of the victim is unknown or unknowable. Thus, when the therapist is confronted with a patient who threatens another but who refuses to say who that person is and the therapist cannot guess the person's identity or where the patient expresses a desire to discharge a weapon into a crowd (in which case the potential victims cannot be known), the therapist will hospitalize or take some other action.

Efficacy. The primary reason for warning is still to protect third parties, not just to prevent potential liability. To date, only one study bears directly on the efficacy of warning to prevent violence. Beck (1982) has reported a small series in which he used warning; following warning, no violence occurred. However, the study was uncontrolled: Beck did not first decide to warn, then randomly warn some potential victims and not others to ascertain whether warning affected the outcome. At present, then, the data supporting warning are extremely limited. Nevertheless, the absence of data should not be misconstrued as implying that therapists should always employ clinical interventions in preference to warning. One point of Beck's article (1982) was that he had used warning therapeutically to confront patients about the real-world consequences of their behavior; thus, the warning–protecting dichotomy may be a false one.

To confound matters, there is persuasive, albeit anecdotal, evidence that warning may have little effect. *Jablonski* v. *United States* (1983) presents this perspective most dramatically. In that case, the victim and common-law spouse of the murderer knew that her husband had recently attempted to assault her mother sexually. When her mother did not press charges and solicited the aid of the police in obtaining treatment for Jablonski, the victim escorted her spouse to a local hospital. On at least two occasions, the victim spoke with the evaluating psychiatrist, who told her that her husband needed to be in the hospital. The husband refused, and the physicians mistakenly believed that his behavior did not satisfy the statutory grounds for civil commitment (see generally, Shah, 1975). Further, the victim was told that her hus- was dangerous. However, she was not formally warned that continuing to live with him constituted a grave risk to her well-being. Her priest was so concerned for her safety that he insisted that she separate from him, which she did.

Whether or not the discussions that the victim had with the physicians to whom she spoke (she talked with another psychiatrist as well as with the one evaluating Jablonski) or the priest constituted a warning in the technical sense, she knew from her mother's experience, from her own, and from the discussions that Jablonski was dangerous. In this case, then, it is difficult, although not impossible, to believe that a formal warning would have influenced the outcome of events (Mills, 1984b).

This history—Jablonski murdered his common-law spouse when she returned to their apartment on what was intended to be a brief errand—suggests that there is reason to believe that warning will not prevent some violent acts. As an aside, the victim in *Tarasoff* itself had apparently (Winslade and Ross, 1983) been warned repeatedly by her parents to stay away from Poddar, her murderer (*People* v. *Poddar,* 1972). Further, her brother, who had roomed with Poddar, knew of Poddar's obsession with his sister. Again, the events cast doubt on the prophylactic value of warning.

Expanding the Duties

Given a desire to protect third parties from foreseeable violence, it should be evident that linking the duty to protect with warning may not make sense. Nevertheless, there are circumstances in which warning makes considerable sense. In order to develop this point, one needs to be familar with the legal perspectives that underpinned *Tarasoff* and that have supported the subsequent case law.

Essentially, the courts have wanted to ensure that, when an individual who is in the position to hear intimate disclosures anticipates a violent act, the individual behaves to forestall that act. In the abstract, relatively few would quarrel with the notion that, when reasonable, members of society should act to diminish violence. The question is, To whom should the duty extend? When should it vest? How should it be discharged?

Presumably, the courts have hoped to accomplish at least two ends. First, by creating a duty, they underscored the importance of attempting to reduce violence: When one is seriously in doubt, one should act by attempting to protect the intended victim. Second, they wished to recompense the hapless victim. It should be evident that imposing liability broadly increases the likelihood that adequate compensation will be found for the victim.

Limited Liability. Why, then, did the courts not create such broad liability? Several reasons can be adduced: First, courts tend to be conservative and to rule in as narrow a manner as possible. Second, broad changes in the law are nominally the prerogative of the legislative branch of government; however, consider *Brown* v. *Board of Education:* This canon is sometimes violated. Third, courts attempt to articulate a strong rationale when creating a new duty. In *Tarasoff,* the rationale was that the special nature of the psychotherapeutic relationship made certain disclosures more likely to occur and that psychotherapists had historically held themselves out as having expertise in assessing an individual's state of mind.

But, does that rationale make sense? Are there not other relationships in which intimate disclosures are likely? The cleric routinely hears intimate details of people's lives. Where the penitent is relatively devout, the amount and veracity of the material disclosed may be fully comparable to the material disclosed in therapy. Judging by the complex case law of the exclusionary rule — a rule that denies prosecutors certain evidence in order to ensure that coercion is not used — the police routinely learn many details about the lives of detainees, suspects, and prisoners. Further, one might suspect that the police would be at least as good as therapists at predicting violent behavior. (Monahan [1981] suggests that there are insufficient data to support the contention that any one profession is better at predicting violent behavior than any other.) Because of the ironclad rules protecting attorney–client privilege, attorneys learn about their clients' lives in considerable detail. Similar arguments could be made about administrators, employers, judges, parole and probation officers, physicians in general, and teachers. In certain contexts, there is a considerable likelihood that, acting in their official capacity, persons in each of these groups could learn information about future violent behavior.

Given the amount of violence in society, a reasonable person might well argue that *Tarasoff* should be extended legislatively to each of these groups and perhaps to others as well. One difficulty with such an argument, however, is that most of these groups have no formal training in clinical management. Thus, the kinds of clinically oriented strategems (Tardiff, 1981a; Tardiff, 1981b; Tupin, 1983) just outlined for dealing with potentially violent patients are inapplicable. This, then, would be a prototype for situations in which warning is appropriate. When an individual without clinical training believes, by virtue of acting in an official capacity, that another is going to commit a violent act, that individual should make a reasonable effort to notify the relevant law enforcement officials and the potential victim, where the potential victim's identity is known.

Caveats. Some caveats are important. Where an individual does not have clinical training, warning is the only readily available alternative. This may also be true of some who have clinical training. One of the prerogatives that allows psychiatrists to manage potentially violent patients is the power to civilly commit. In most states (Brakel and Rock, in press; "Developments in the Law," 1974), this power is circumscribed, so that nonpsychiatric physicians or psychologists may not have it. For these clinicians, it may be necessary to warn with somewhat greater frequency.

The problem of whom to warn is intriguing. At present, there seem to be no fully satisfactory alternatives. The police are equipped to deal with crime after it occurs; at best, they identify and bring the perpetrator into custody. They are not well equipped, economically or temperamentally, to perform long-term stakeouts on the off chance of preventing an assault. Given most patients' low base rates for violent behavior, most predictions of future violence will not come true (Monahan, 1981). Moreover, warning the potential victim is not a particularly satisfactory solution. Although Wexler (1979) has dissected the virtues of *Tarasoff* from the victim's viewpoint, the fact remains that, for most potential victims, a warning is quite frightening; perhaps worse, it occurs to little avail, since most predictions of future violence will be false. Most potential victims have neither the inclination nor the resources to hire around-the-clock security forces to protect them. This does not mean, however, that the potential victim will not feel some relief in knowing that he or she can avoid the potential perpetrator or that the potential victim does not have a moral right to know that he or she is potentially at risk. When possible, it would seem that warning both the police and the potential victim is the best alternative. Still, warning may do relatively little to diminish the chance that violence will occur, and it may be attended by a relatively high social cost — useless police stakeouts and needless worry on the part of the potential victim.

Social Policy. A comprehensive examination of the complex social equities involved in broadening the duty to third parties is beyond the scope of this chapter. No doubt, many psychotherapists would welcome an extension of the rule both out of social conviction (that everyone should do his or her share to reduce the potential for violence) and out of self-interest (it does not seem fair that only psychotherapists, out of all those who routinely encounter reports of potential violence in the accomplishment of their profession, should be burdened with the *Tarasoff* obligations). On the other hand, most (all?) professions considered here would be reluctant to assume the *Tarasoff* duties. At the risk of appearing to be concerned more with law and order than with civil liberties, I believe that, because violence is pandemic, society should endeavor to create reasonable obligations that tend, in aggregate, to reduce violence. The duty to protect third parties from potentially violent acts appears to be a reasonable obligation; still, as previously noted, the present state of the empirical literature does not establish this point clearly.

From the policy perspective, there is little reason to couple liability with negligence: The law recognizes the concept of strict liability as a way of compensating those who are injured without necessitating a finding of negligence (Levine, 1984). This is an important alternative to the traditional linking of liability, and hence of compensation, with negligence, as it allows injured victims to be compensated even when the professional acts correctly. The difficulties of endeavoring to predict violence in the context of protecting third parties have been discussed elsewhere (Mills, 1984a; Wettstein, 1984). Since the difficulty is great, the technologies are immature (there is no developed paradigm), and professional experience varies widely (particularly if *Tarasoff* duties are extended to other professionals), the creation of strict liability would serve to greatly enhance the economic protection afforded victims. (The imposition of strict liability, however, would both necessarily and significantly increase the cost of psychotherapy, and, during a period when health costs are being scrutinized, one can well wonder about the desirability of such an increase.) Further, such a scheme would not alleviate much violence in society: Most violent acts are not discussed prior to their occurrence with a person acting within the scope of his or her professional duties. American society does not seem ready to require all citizens, irrespective of role or frame of mind, to act to restrain others from violence.

Conclusion

This chapter has presented two viewpoints about the *Tarasoff* line of cases. First, through conscientious clinical practice, professionals can reasonably discharge the duty to protect. Second, from the perspective of protecting society from violence, the duty should be expanded. Since both perspectives are contrary to the conventional wisdom, they both have been elaborated in some detail.

In closing, three points merit underscoring. First, because the effects of warning (both on the patient and on the potential victim) have not been fully studied, warning should not become routine clinical practice until such time as predictions of violence become significantly more accurate. Second, legislative attempts at circumscribing the impact of *Tarasoff* tend to focus excessively on discharging the duty through warning. Third, mental health professionals, their historic claims to the contrary notwithstanding, do not have a *via regia* to predictions of violent behavior; hence, all those who encounter disclosures of future harm in the course of their profession are similarly equipped (psychiatrists' and other professionals' ability to civilly commit is the only example of disparity in this regard) to protect society.

References

Appelbaum, P. S. "The Expansion of Liability for Patients' Violent Acts." *Hospital and Community Psychiatry,* 1984, *35,* 13–14.

Beck, J. C. "When a Patient Threatens Violence: An Empirical Study of Clinical Practice After *Tarasoff.*" *Bulletin of the American Academy of Psychiatry and the Law,* 1982, *10,* 189–201.

Berger, P. A. "The Medical Treatment of Mental Illness." *Science,* 1978, *200,* 974–981.

Brakel, S. J., and Rock, R. S. *The Mentally Disabled and the Law.* (3rd ed.) Chicago: University of Chicago Press, in press.

Brown v. *Board of Education,* 347 U.S. 483, 74 S. Ct. 686 (1954).

Clark v. *New York,* 472 N.Y.S.2d 170 (N.Y. App. Div. 1984).

"Developments in the Law: Civil Commitment of the Mentally Ill." *Harvard Law Review,* 1974, *87,* 1190–1406.

Givelber, D. J., Bowers, W. J., and Blitch, C. L. "*Tarasoff:* Myth and Reality; An Empirical Study of Private Law in Action." *Wisconsin Law Review,* 1984, *2,* 443–497.

Hamilton v. *Reynolds,* 341 N.W.2d 152 (Mich. Ct. App. 1983).

Jablonski v. *United States,* 712 F.2d 391 (9th Cir. 1983)

Kroll, J., and Mackenzie, T. B. "When Psychiatrists Are Liable: Risk Management and Violent Patients." *Hospital and Community Psychiatry,* 1983, *34,* 29–37.

LeBlang, T. R. "Duty to Warn Third Parties Threatened by a Patient." *Legal Aspects of Medical Practice,* 1982, *10* (8), 1–4.

Levine, M. L. Personal communication, March 1984.

Mills, M. J. "The So-Called Duty to Warn: The Psychotherapeutic Duty to Protect Third Parties from Patients' Violent Acts." *Behavioral Sciences and the Law,* 1984a, *2,* 237-258.

Mills, M. J. "The *Tarasoff* Duties Expand—*Jablonski* and *Hedlund.*" *American Academy of Psychiatry and the Law Newsletter,* 1984b, *9* (1), 8-11.

Monahan, J. *The Clinical Prediction of Violent Behavior.* Department of Health and Human Services No. (ADM)81-921. Rockville, Md.: National Institute of Mental Health, 1981.

People v. *Poddar,* 103 Cal. Rptr. 84(1972). See also the California Supreme Court's subsequent reversal at 10 Cal. 3d 750, 518 P.2d 342 (1974).

Roth, L. H. "Dangerousness, Confidentiality, and the Duty to Warn." *American Journal of Psychiatry,* 1977, *134,* 508-511.

Runch, B. "Survey Shows Therapists Misunderstood *Tarasoff* Rule." *Hospital and Community Psychiatry,* 1984, *35,* 429-430.

Shah, S. A. "Dangerousness and Civil Commitment of the Mentally Ill: Some Public Policy Considerations." *American Journal of Psychiatry,* 1975, *132,* 501-505.

Slovenko, R. "Psychotherapy and Confidentiality." *Cleveland State Law Review,* 1975, *24,* 375-391.

Stone, A. A. "Suing Psychotherapists to Safeguard Society." *Harvard Law Review,* 1976, *90,* 358-378.

Tarasoff v. *Regents of the University of California,* 118 Cal. Rptr. 129, 529 P.2d 533 (1974), reargued, 17 Cal. 3d 425, 551 P.2d 334 (1976).

Tardiff, K. "Assaults in Hospitals and Placement in the Community." *Bulletin of the American Academy of Psychiatry and the Law,* 1981a, *9,* 33-39.

Tardiff, K. "Emergency Control Measures for Psychiatric Inpatients." *Journal of Nervous and Mental Disease,* 1981b, *169,* 614-618.

Tupin, J. P. "The Violent Patient: A Strategy of Management and Diagnosis." *Hospital and Community Psychiatry,* 1983, *34,* 37-40.

Wettstein, R. M. "The Prediction of Violent Behavior and the Duty to Protect Third Parties." *Behavioral Sciences and the Law,* 1984, *2,* 291-318.

Wexler, D. B. "Patients, Therapists, and Third Parties: The Victimologicl Virtues of *Tarasoff.*" *International Journal of Law and Psychiatry,* 1979, *2,* 1-28.

Whalen v. *Nevada,* No. 14457 (Nev. Sup. Ct. Jan. 25, 1984).

Winslade, W. J., and Ross, J. R. *The Insanity Defense.* New York: Scribner's, 1983.

*Mark J. Mills is chief, Psychiatry Service, West Los Angeles Veterans
Administration Medical Center, Brentwood Division; director, Program
in Psychiatry and Law, Neuropsychiatric Institute and Clinics; and associate
professor, Department of Psychiatry and Biobehavioral Sciences, University
of California at Los Angeles.*

*What is happening to psychiatric confidentiality must be understood
in terms of shifting values and priorities in society at large.*

The Erosion of Psychiatric Confidentiality

Ben Bursten

Psychiatric confidentiality is the subject of much debate and uncertainty.
Rachlin and Applebaum (1983) have pointed out that legal decisions are coming so rapidly and inconsistently that the practicing psychiatrist is hard-
pressed to grasp the rules of the game. In today's world of image and illusion,
it is sometimes hard to know whether a particular regulation promotes or
erodes confidentiality. Slovenko (1974) said that psychiatric privilege laws are
so full of holes that they are virtually useless. Nye (1980) analyzed four bills in
Congress that purported to protect the privacy of medical records; she showed
that all four bills widened, rather than narrowed, divulgence.

Whether in fact a past in which patient confidentiality was guaranteed
ever existed, we now feel that even the ideal of confidentiality is slipping from
our grasp. In order to understand what is happening and where we might be
going, we must review some of the basic issues.

Justifying Confidentiality

Psychiatric confidentiality has been justified on four grounds: respect
for the individual, the dangers of stigma, constitutional guarantees, and the
state's interest in promoting the healing enterprise.

S. Rachlin (Ed.). *Legal Encroachment on Psychiatric Practice.* New Directions for
Mental Health Services, no. 25. San Francisco: Jossey-Bass, March 1985.

Respect for the Individual. The concept of respect for the individual is invoked with almost mystical reverence when we refer in the abstract to psychiatric ethics and in the historical concrete to the Hippocratic oath. Neither is binding, and both are used as rhetorical arguments by some who have neither read the former nor sworn the latter. Respect for the individual does not flow from great principles; it comes from within. It is lacking in psychiatrists who talk about patients, laugh about patients, or treat patients impersonally as part of a caseload.

Basically, respect for the individual is the concept or feeling that each individual has worth because he or she is a person and that the "boundaries" which define that individual must not be breached or weakened against the person's wishes except under the most compelling circumstances. To me, this is the one unrebuttable justification for psychiatric confidentiality. Unfortunately, because it is a value, it is also unsupportable; one either assigns it high priority, or one does not.

The Dangers of Stigma. A stigma may be attached to being a psychiatric patient (Beigler, 1979; Lanman, 1980). The possibility is well illustrated by the case of Senator Thomas Eagleton, whose career as a vice-presidential candidate came to an abrupt end with the exposure of his previous psychiatric history. I have personally known people in politics who acknowledged that they were suffering and wanted psychiatric treatment but who felt they could not afford the risk of disclosure. Many of us have had patients who paid cash and declined insurance benefits because they feared being stigmatized. The stigma is not necessarily confined to the middle and upper socioeconomic classes. During the early 1960s, I had the opportunity to work in an alcoholism clinic that accepted court-ordered referrals. Quite a few potential patients never showed up. They preferred to serve time in the workhouse, which was less stigmatizing in their community. Beyond the stigma imposed by being a psychiatric patient, there are the dangers of specific divulgences about one's thoughts, opinions, and especially about one's feelings toward others, which could have unfortunate repercussions if revealed.

Constitutional Guarantees. The sociopolitical reflection of respect for the individual was important to the founding fathers. They wanted to make sure that the rights of individual citizens would not be trampled on by an oppressive government. However, nowhere in the Constitution is the right of privacy (let alone the right of psychiatric confidentiality) spelled out. A constitutional right of privacy had been implied by the courts, but it was not until *Griswold* v. *Connecticut* (1965) that the Supreme Court specifically declared it. Just how many types of individual activity fall within the zone of privacy that is constitutionally protected is not at all clear (*Carey* v. *Population Services International,* 1977). With regard to medical information that may reflect adversely on a patient's character, the Supreme Court (*Whalen* v. *Roe,* 1977, p. 605) said that it "arguably has its roots in the Constitution." Subsequently, some lower courts (*In re B.,* 1978; *Hawaii Psychiatric Society District Branch of the American*

Psychiatric Association v. *Aryioshi,* 1979) have rendered the opinion that psychiatric confidences may be constitutionally protected.

Smith (1980) has argued that psychotherapeutic confidentiality should fall within the zone of privacy protected by the constitution. He maintained that mental illness can disrupt family life and interfere with one's ability to exercise religious beliefs, speech, and press. Since these fundamental interests are guaranteed by our Constitution, those enterprises that enable us to realize them should be protected. Smith's arguments were recently incorporated into a decision of the Sixth Circuit (*In re Zanuga,* 1983); during the same year, the Seventh Circuit Court reiterated that a psychotherapist–patient privilege is "arguable" (*In re Pebsworth,* 1983, p. 263).

The State's Interest in the Healing Enterprise. While the health of citizens is not a constitutional right, both historically and as a matter of fact the government has had an interest in promoting the health and welfare of the populace and in minimizing impediments to health. The first doctor–patient confidentiality law in the United States (2 N. Y. Rev. Stat., 1829, p. 406) was said to promote health in two ways. In the first place, patients must be able to tell their doctor everything in order to obtain proper treatment. In the second place, if the patients fear subsequent disclosure, they will be deterred from going to the doctor altogether. It is obvious that these arguments apply to the psychiatric enterprise, and they have been reiterated by current commentators (Lanman, 1980; Nye, 1980). Smith (1980) has compiled a list of about thirty articles supporting the view that confidentiality is essential to effctive psychotherapy and that, without it, people will stay away. The trust that people put in their doctors, which allows types of intimacies not usually found in other enterprises, is called a *fiduciary relationship,* and doctors are at risk of violating this relationship if they reveal confidences (*Horne* v. *Patton,* 1973). At the present time, there is a hodgepodge of state laws, some protecting doctor–patient confidentiality, some protecting psychotherapeutic confidentiality, and some protecting psychiatric confidentiality.

The federal government has promoted health by passing an alcohol and drug treatment law that quite strictly protects the confidentiality of information in federally funded programs (42 U.S.C.A. sec. 290dd-3). Congress was well aware that nonconfidentiality would keep many abusers away. However, it would be naive to believe that Congress was concerned only with the health of abusers. The lawmakers were reacting to the moral connotations of abuse and to the economic and safety costs of the associated crime (Lanman, 1980). Beigler (1980) tried to blend health and nonhealth arguments to promote psychotherapeutic confidentiality in treatment generally, not just in treatment of substance abuse. He states that, in addition to improving patients' health, therapy promoted the integrity of the family and rendered people less dangerous to society. However, these arguments have not been persuasive to legislatures. Confidentiality is not as well protected in psychotherapy as it is in alcohol and drug programs.

The Justifications Rebutted

Respect for the Individual. Reliance on such principles as the Hippocratic oath to support the concept of human dignity and respect has undermined this powerful justification. The Hippocratic oath is no longer sacrosanct. Such commentators as Schuchman (1980) have pointed out that the medical enterprise was much simpler 2,400 years ago than it is today. Nowadays, the dyadic model of medicine is rare; in 1975, allied health workers provided 95 percent of the direct health care in the United States, and two thirds of the services were paid for by third parties (Parmut, 1981). Hippocrates could not possibly have foreseen the complexity of modern health care. Furthermore, up to a few centuries ago, medicine, mysticism, and religion were closely bound (Sigerist, 1941). The ethics of one was the ethics of the other. However, the situation has changed. As medicine becomes more complex, its ethical base may shift. There is no expectation that the scientist or the businessman will hold to the ethical standards of the priest. Thus, respect for the individual as a justification for psychiatric confidentiality must stand alone rather than lean on "authorities." To my mind, it is a powerful and unrebuttable justification.

The Dangers of Stigma. The fact that increasing numbers of people have come for treatment over the last few decades suggests that the stigma may be lessening. At the same time, people who are ashamed to seek treatment might shun it even if confidentiality were guaranteed. The modern medical office building is heavily frequented, and it is relatively easy for others to see one walking in and out of an office or sitting in a waiting room. Absence from usual activities to keep doctor appointments must be explained. One might argue that, where stigma exists, no statute or policy can eradicate it. This, of course, is debatable.

Constitutional Guarantees. Even if the courts should ultimately decide unequivocally that psychiatrist–patient confidentiality is a constitutionally protected aspect of the right of privacy, no right is absolute. The courts must still evaluate how significant or important a right is. Basic or fundamental rights may be abridged only when the competing state interest is compelling (*Roe* v. *Wade,* 1973). Thus, even if psychiatrist–patient confidentiality were constitutionally protected, two other factors would enter into the degree of protection: First, how important or fundamental is this right? Second, how important is the state's competing interest in divulgence? Here, the situation is very fluid, and these competing state interests comprise what is seen as the attack on and erosion of confidentiality. We shall consider these interests later in this chapter.

Even if psychiatrist–patient confidentiality were constitutionally protected, not all aspects would need to be afforded the same degree of protection. There are levels of psychiatric information, and some courts are recognizing that the state's interests can be satisfied by the divulgence of certain information, while other information remains confidential. In *In re Zanuga* (1983) and

In re Pebsworth (1983), the courts distinguished basic logistical information necessary for auditing from accounts of psychotherapeutic discussions. I can visualize four levels of information divulgence: no divulgence whatsoever; verification of attendance, billing, diagnosis, and treatment modality; divulgence of the patient's reports of his or her actions; and divulgence of the patient's reports of his or her thoughts and feelings.

The State's Interest in the Healing Enterprise. I have never seen arguments against the state's interest in health, although disagreements about how far the government should go to support such interest are frequent. Since there is no constitutional demand on the government to provide medical care (*Maher* v. *Roe,* 1977), it can pick and choose which services it wishes to provide (*Dandridge* v. *Williams,* 1970).

Although the state may have an interest in fostering psychiatric health care, not everyone has agreed that absolute confidentiality is necessary in order to achieve this purpose. The California Supreme Court (*In re Lifschutz,* 1970) noted that psychotherapeutic practice has flourished despite the exceptions to confidentiality. Wechsler (1979) has pointed out that confidentiality can be countertherapeutic in dangerous situations. Miller (1981) has suggested that, for the interests of both the patient and the state, confidentiality should be abridged for committed patients when it is necessary to ensure continuity of care. There is relatively little disagreement with the notion that suicidal psychotic people should lose their confidentiality when divulgence is necessary to hospitalize them. It is probably fair to say that confidentiality may be necessary in certain cases and not in others. The problem is that we do not know in advance in which cases it is necessary, nor do we know the scope of the divulgence that may ultimately be demanded.

From a public rather than an individual health standpoint, some segments of organized psychiatry (Altman, 1981; Penner, 1981) have argued that furnishing data to third-party payers makes psychiatric treatment more available to those who need it. And, researchers, such as Robins (1978) and Wing (1981), emphasize the health benefits to be reaped by research that involves disclosures to scientists. In an attempt to guard the patient population against mentally ill physicians, many states now require the applicant for licensure to divulge his or her past psychiatric history. The American Psychiatric Association (1984) has taken the position that coerced disclosure of physicians' past psychiatric records should not be allowed.

Competing Interests

The health interests that compete with confidentiality cluster chiefly around third-party payment and have to do with regulation and accountability. Whether public or private, a third-party payer has a stake in setting down certain rules for the operation of enterprises for which it is willing to pay. Parmut (1981) has pointed out that not only must claims be substantiated, but information is necessary for fiscal planning and for innovation in the methods of delivering health care and in scientific technique. The U.S. Supreme Court (*Whalen* v. *Roe,* 1977) declared that limited disclosure of information from medical records is allowable for purposes of regulation and accountability. Guilette (1981) has said that divulgence is necessary in order for third-party payers to know that the claims relate only to conditions for which they have contracted to pay, although Slovenko (1975) and others have indicated that this interest in divulgence may be undercut by the misinformation that psychiatrists sometimes put on the forms in order to protect their patients. Both Slovenko (1979) and Stone (1981) have pointed out that divulgence may be necessary to detect fraud and poor treatment. Some courts (*Hawaii Psychiatric Society* v. *Aryioshi,* 1979; *In re Zanuga,* 1983; *In re Pebsworth,* 1983) have agreed that certain needs of third-party payers outweigh the need for confidentiality, but they have tended to set narrow limits on just what kinds of material need to be divulged. There might be less concern about giving information to third-party payers if one could be certain that the divulgence would stop there. However, Beigler (1979) and Rosner (1980) have cited instances of serious leaks by insurance companies, and Sharfstein and others (1980) have pointed out that the laws governing divulgence of insurance information are unpredictably subject to change. This fact is brought home forcefully by the disclosure that the General Services Administration is currently negotiating contracts giving federal agencies around-the-clock access to the files of credit agencies, which have millions of records, and that these agencies have wide network linkages to give and receive information (Burnham, 1984).

There are other societal interests that compete with confidentiality and that may more directly counter the patient's interests or desires. Society has a strong interest in the protection and welfare of children, particularly because they are unable to care for or to defend themselves. Some courts have ruled that confidentiality regarding parents must give way to the infant's need in custody disputes (*Shaffer* v. *Spicer,* 1974) and that the need to report child abuse supersedes psychotherapeutic confidentiality (*People* v. *Stritzinger,* 1983). Indeed, a court just ruled that even the strictly controlled confidentiality of alcohol programs may have to yield to the need to prosecute child molesters (*Minnesota* v. *Audring,* 1984). Even the American Psychiatric Association (1979) has made an exception to confidentiality in the case of child abuse.

One of the most publicized competing interests of the past decade was that of the patient–litigant exception. The courts (*In re Lifschutz,* 1970; *Caesar* v. *Montanos,* 1976) stated that, when a plaintiff claims that his or her mental state resulted from the actions of another person, the interests of justice require some access to the plaintiff's psychiatric records. And, in the criminal sphere, courts have ruled that limited divulgence is mandatory in cases involving fraud against third-party payers (*Hawaii Psychiatric Society* v. *Aryioshi,* 1979; *In re Zanuga,* 1983) and that psychiatric data may be compelled if necessary to impeach the credibility of one accusing a defendant (*In re Pittsburgh Action Against*

Rape, 1981). Even Smith (1980)—a staunch advocate of psychotherapeutic confidentiality—made exceptions in criminal cases where divulgence was necessary to impeach witnesses or accusers.

Perhaps the most concern has been raised about prosecutors and investigators seeking psychiatric information in order to build a criminal case against a patient (Nye, 1980). Data kept in federal agencies are available to investigators for criminal prosecution purposes (5 U.S.C.A. sec. 552a(b)(7)). Some courts have taken the position that the need for criminal prosecutions may override psychiatric confidentiality (*General Motors Corporation* v. *Director of National Institute of Occupational Safety and Health,* 1980). The competing interest here is the government's police power to preserve order and safety. When safety is threatened by physical danger, the pressure for divulgence is very high. Psychiatrists do not hesitate to protect society by hospitalizing psychotic patients who may be dangerous, and, if confidentiality must be breached, so be it. We may hesitate to warn potential victims, however, as Mills notes in Chapter Six. And, when it comes to exposing past offenders (who may become future offenders), psychiatrists most often object to divulgence. Criminal investigative agencies, whose agendas lie more in the area of safety than in the area of health, are always pressing to get information that might help them.

Where Will It All End?

The interests and counterinterests, the requirements for confidentiality and the demands for divulgence have created a patchwork of laws, regulations, and court decisions that would baffle a legal scholar, let alone your average working psychiatrist. What happened to the good old days when psychiatrists were only agents of their patients?

What happened is that the old days, while good for the doctor because there was less regulation, were probably never as good for the patients as we like to think they were. We were never solely agents of our patients, as Szasz (1964) pointed out two decades ago. Doctors have always been members of society, having connections and obligations that extended to employers, schools, the military, and even the police and communicating with these others whenever they thought it wise to do so. What has changed is that patients are no longer as timorous as they once were. They are no longer as convinced that everything we do under the guise of being their agent is really in their best interest. They and their lawyers are beginning to ask, If you are supposed to be my agent, how can you use medical discretion to override my discretion? While such overriding has occurred more in other areas than in confidentiality, the net effect is that the magic of the medical relationship has been weakened in the public eye, and the information seekers have become more vociferous. This tendency has been abetted by the many forces attempting to discredit psychiatry (Dietz, 1977).

Society is becoming hungry for information (Naisbitt, 1984). Our technology and our health enterprise support systems are now much more complex; increasingly, delivery of service requires a network, and networks require communication. Again, the magical medical relationship, the trusted dyad, is broken. Further, our information technology has improved; as it has become physically miniaturized, it has greatly increased in scope and capability. I think that the information trend is inevitable; when human beings have technology, they will use it, and morals will be refashioned.

What happened is that psychiatry is changing. In the first place, since there are more of us, and we are better organized, we are more visible, and more people want what we know. In the second place, as psychiatric technology advances, some within our profession demean the person by attempting to draw a line between what they call "real disease" and "problems in living." (I will not cite references: You know who you are!) As attempts to invalidate psychotherapy as a bona fide medical enterprise continue, we shall see a further weakening of the dyad and of the confidentiality that goes along with the fiduciary relationship. In the third place, psychiatry, along with the rest of medicine, has become big business, and its escalating costs are now being underwritten by third parties. Any business in which the consumer is not the payer is particularly open to fraud if access to records is limited. In the fourth place, the endangered economic position of psychiatry, together with the complexities of health delivery systems, have already changed our official view of psychiatric confidentiality from one of complete confidentiality, except where we reveal what we feel is in the interest of the individual patient, to a notion of confidentiality as whatever is needed to make provision of our services ecoomically feasible. In the fifth place, we have new research technologies and methodologies that were unavailable a few decades ago. I predict that the psychiatrists now being trained under the conditions of tomorrow will generally be less concerned about patient confidentiality than their predecessors.

What happened is that the past two decades have seen a shift in public and governmental interest away from health and welfare and toward public order and safety. This does not mean that psychiatric confidentiality has lessened. It means that the direction from which demands for information come will shift from health agencies to police agencies. Even pressures for auditing and accountability will probably decrease as the profession gradually moves toward the private and uninsured sector, and there is less to audit and regulate.

What happened is that there has been a shift away from privacy in society in general, not just in psychiatry. The paper and computer trails that we leave in the course of our activities, which would have horrified people fifty years ago, are now taken in stride. The social security card is now the nation's identity card. Pressures for divulgence of census and income tax information would shock those who originally set up these systems.

It is always dangerous to make predictions. The best I can do is to point out that the future of psychiatric confidentiality has less to do with psychiatry than it does with society at large. We are talking about competing interests, competing values. At bottom, we are probably talking about several conflicting themes. To what extent is our society willing to subordinate respect for the individual to public and social needs? What priority will we give to health enterprises? What priority will we give to public order and safety, to efficiency or commercial interests?

One thing should be made clear. The legal confusion surrounding psychiatric practice is not unique to our enterprise; we are not being picked on. If you think that our situation is ambiguous, ask any manufacturer about product liability or environmental protection rulings. Consumerism, legal militancy, and changing values reflect the times in which we live. Although we may long for the past, when psychiatric confidentiality was a relatively settled issue, we are both the products and the agents of the changing times of today. It would be naive to think that we can conserve psychiatric confidentiality if we do not oppose other societal erosions of privacy. We do not have that kind of clout as a special interest. Society is shifting from a focus on the individual to perceived societal needs, and psychiatry is drifting with the tide. Whether this is good or bad depends on your point of view.

References

Altman, H. G. "Confidentiality Safeguards and Psychiatric Care." *American Journal of Psychiatry,* 1981, *138,* 120.

American Psychiatric Association. "Model Law on Confidentiality of Health and Social Service Records." *American Journal of Psychiatry,* 1979, *136,* 138–144.

American Psychiatric Association. "Position Statement on Confidentiality of Medical Records: Does the Physician Have a Right to Privacy Concerning His or Her Own Health Records?" *American Journal of Psychiatry,* 1984, *141,* 331–332.

Beigler, J. S. "Statement of the American Psychiatric Association Before the Subcommittee on Government Information and Individual Rights." *New York State Journal of Medicine,* 1979, *79,* 2088–2092.

Beigler, J. S. "Psychiatric Confidentiality and the American Legal System: An Ethical Conflict." In S. Bloch and P. Chodoff (Eds.), *Psychiatric Ethics.* Oxford, England: Oxford University Press, 1980.

Burnham, D. "U.S. Agencies to Get Direct Link to Credit Records." *New York Times,* April 8, 1984, p. 23.

Caesar v. *Montanos,* 542 F. 2d 1064 (9th Cir. 1976).

Carey v. *Population Services International,* 431 U.S. 678 (1977).

Dandridge v. *Williams,* 397 U.S. 471 (1970).

Dietz, P. E. "Social Discrediting of Psychiatry: The Prostasis of Legal Disfranchisement." *American Journal of Psychiatry,* 1977, *134,* 1356–1360.

General Motors Corporation v. *Director of National Institute of Occupational Safety and Health,* 636 F. 2d 163 (6th Cir. 1980).

Griswold v. *Connecticut,* 381 U.S. 479 (1965).

Guilette, W. "Letter to the Editor." *Hastings Center Reports,* 1981, *11,* 44.

Hawaii Psychiatric Society District Branch of the American Psychiatric Association v. *Aryioshi,* 481 F. Supp. 1028 (D. Hawaii 1979).

Horne v. *Patton,* 287 So. 2d 824 (Ala. 1973).

In re B., 394 A. 2d 419 (Pa. 1978).

In re Lifschutz, 467 P. 2d 557 (Cal. 1970).

In re Pebsworth, 705 F. 2d 261 (7th Cir. 1983).

In re Pittsburgh Action Against Rape, 49 U.S.L.W. 2500 (Pa. Sup. Ct. Jan. 23, 1981).

In re Zanuga, 714 F. 2d 632 (6th Cir. 1983).

Lanman, R. B. "The Federal Confidentiality Protection for Alcohol and Drug Abuse Patient Records: A Model for Mental Health and Other Medical Records?" *American Journal of Orthopsychiatry,* 1980, *50,* 666–677.

Maher v. *Roe,* 432 U.S. 464 (1977).

Miller, R. D. "Confidentiality or Communication in the Treatment of the Mentally Ill." *Bulletin of the American Academy of Psychiatry and the Law,* 1981, *9,* 54–59.

Minnesota v. *Audring,* 52 U.S.L.W. 2425 (Minn. Sup. Ct. Jan. 13, 1984.)

Naisbitt, J. *Megatrends.* New York: Warner Books, 1984.

N. Y. Rev. Stat., 1829, p. 406.

Nye, S. G. "Patient Confidentiality and Privacy." *American Journal of Orthopsychiatry,* 1980, *50,* 649–658.

Parmut, W. "Public Health Protection and the Privacy of Medical Records." *Harvard Civil Rights–Civil Liberties Law Review,* 1981, *10,* 265–304.

Penner, N. R. "Letter to the Editor." *Hastings Center Reports,* 1981, *11,* 43–44.

People v. *Stritzinger,* 668 P. 2d 738 (Cal. 1983).

Rachlin, S., and Appelbaum, P. S. "The Limits of Confidentiality." *Hospital and Community Psychiatry,* 1983, *34,* 589–590.

Robins, L. "Privacy Regulations and Longitudinal Studies." Paper presented to the American Association for the Advancement of Science, Washington, D. C., February 1978.

Roe v. *Wade,* 410 U.S. 113 (1973).

Rosner, B. L. "Psychiatry, Confidentiality, and Insurance Claims." *Hastings Center Reports,* 1980, *10,* 5–7.

Schuchman, H. "Confidentiality: Practice Issues in New Legislation." *American Journal of Orthopsychiatry,* 1980, *50,* 641–648.

Shaffer v. *Spicer,* 215 N.W. 2d 134 (S. D. 1974).

Sharfstein, S. S., Towery, O. B., and Milowe, I. D. "Accuracy of Diagnostic Information Submitted to an Insurance Company." *American Journal of Psychiatry,* 1980, *137,* 70–73.

Sigerist, H. E. *Medicine and Human Welfare.* New Haven, Conn.: Yale University Press, 1941.

Slovenko, R. "Psychotherapist–Patient Testimonial Privilege: A Picture of Misguided Hope." *Catholic University Law Review,* 1974, *23,* 649–673.

Slovenko, R. "Psychotherapy and Confidentiality." *Cleveland State Law Review,* 1975, *24,* 375–396.

Slovenko, R. "Accountability and the Abuse of Confidentiality in the Practice of Psychiatry." *International Journal Law and Psychiatry,* 1979, *2,* 431–454.

Smith, S. R. "Constitutional Privacy in Psychotherapy." *George Washington Law Review,* 1980, *49,* 1–60.

Stone, A. A. "Letter to the Editor." *Hastings Center Reports,* 1981, *11,* 44–45.

Szasz, T. S. "The Psychiatrist as Double Agent." *Trans-Action,* 1964, *4,* 16–23.

Wechsler, D. B. "Patients, Therapists, and Third Parties: The Victimological Virtues of *Tarasoff.*" *International Journal of Law and Psychiatry,* 1979, *2,* 1–28.

Whalen v. *Roe,* 429 U.S. 589 (1977).

Wing, J. "Ethics and Psychiatric Research." In S. Bloch and P. Chodoff (Eds.) *Psychiatric Ethics.* Oxford, England: Oxford University Press, 1981.

Ben Bursten in professor of psychiatry, University of Tennessee College of Medicine, Memphis.

*The trend toward increasing patients' access to their own mental
health records has changed charting practices and influenced patient
care, with mixed results.*

Patient Access to Mental Health Records: Impact on Clinical Practice

Harold I. Schwartz
Stephen Rachlin

The medical record has traditionally been considered the property of the physician or the hospital. Within the last decade, however, this situation has been changing rapidly, as more and more states have enacted legislation that grants patients the right of access to their records. A recent California statute (California Health and Safety Code, 1984) goes so far as to provide for the possible suspension or revocation of the license of any health care provider who fails to comply.

The position that a medical or mental health record is the sole property of the clinician has proven vulnerable to the argument that the patient has a property right, if not to the actual record, then to the information that it contains. Clinicians are being required to adjust to a change in practice in the service of what is gradually being established as a new right. The American Psychiatric Association (1979) added momentum to this trend by publishing a model law promoting the prerogative of mental patients to have access to their records.

The concept of a license to review and possess one's mental health record placed a number of values in conflict. It may be useful to look at how

80

we arrived at this juncture and to examine just what we know about the impact that patient access to mental health records can have on patients and on practice.

Social and Legal Trends Leading to Access Laws

The developments that, taken together, establish and empower a right follow many paths. On the federal level, the Truth in Lending Act, the Fair Credit Reporting Act, the Freedom of Information Act, and the Privacy Act all increased citizens' access to various types of records. The consumer movement of the 1960s and 1970s left the public with a new sense of its rights with regard to the purchase of all products and services. Certainly, medicine and psychiatry have been undergoing a deidealization in the public eye, which has led to demands for increased accountability and for increased patient autonomy within the doctor–patient relationship. In the mental health field, legal advocacy of patients' rights has affected civil commitment, standards of treatment in both public and private facilities, and the right to refuse treatment, to name only three areas. The issue of patients' access to their records can be seen as a logical extension of the advocacy of patients' rights in general and of the doctrine of informed consent in particular, combined with a heightened sensitivity to issues of confidentiality.

Anthony (1977) and Tucker (1978) have reviewed the evolution of court decisions that have taken us from the view of records as the sole property of doctors or hospitals to the present view that the patient has a limited property right in the record. The most frequently cited case involving a psychiatric patient is *Gotkin* v. *Miller* (1974). Janet Gotkin was voluntarily hospitalized several times between 1962 and 1970. In 1973, after contracting to write a book about Janet's experiences, the Gotkins requested copies of her records from the three New York hospitals involved. The requests were refused. The Gotkins then filed a class action suit claiming that refusals to allow access to the record violated the federal constitutional rights of former mental patients. The lower court granted the defendants' motion for summary judgment, holding that there was no genuine issue of fact to be decided. The Second Circuit Court of Appeals, in upholding this decision, found no constitutionally protected property interest in unrestricted access to the psychiatric records in question and that any such right that might exist had to be defined by state law.

State legislatures have indeed been active in delineating the degree to which records are available. As recently as 1965, only a few states had access laws that defined current or former patients' rights to review and copy their records without resorting to litigation, and charts of mental patients were often treated more restrictively than other medical records. The 1973 report of the secretary's Commission on Medical Malpractice (U.S. Department of Health, Education, and Welfare, 1973) added further impetus by concluding that patients had a right of access to the information contained in their records and by recommending that states should statutorily enable this end. Madden (1982) reports that fourteen jurisdictions have statutes bearing on a patient's right of access to his or her medical records. Two of these statutes refer only to mental health records, two specifically exempt mental health records, and the others are quite variable in scope, detail, and extent. In addition, other states permit patient inspection of records via confidentiality or freedom of information laws.

Partially in recognition of these developments, the American Psychiatric Association (1979) published its model law on confidentiality of health and social service records, which clearly supported the right of mental patients to see and copy their records. Somehow, that recommendation has received comparatively little attention. The proposal would allow a patient to challenge the "accuracy, completeness or relevancy" of the record and to add a corrective statement if necessary. Restrictions on the principle of general access are spelled out. The service provider may withhold the record if he or she feels that disclosure would be detrimental to the patient. In such cases, the patient must be advised of his or her right to appoint another clinician of his or her choice as a "clinical mediator"; the clinical mediator reviews the record and independently decides whether or not to release it to the patient. If the patient remains dissatisfied, he or she has a right to petition for judicial review and court order. Further, the model law stipulates that minors twelve years old or over must consent in writing to the release of their records to their parents. A special provision is made for "personal notes." These are not to be accessible to the patient, and they may contain confidential information imparted by third parties, material revealed by the patient that would be injurious to his or her relationships with others, and the therapist's own "speculations, impressions, hunches, and reminders."

Studies of Patient Access to Records

Although the legislative trend toward increased access is unmistakable, and the American Psychiatric Association and others have taken an affirmative position, the fact remains that our knowledge of the actual impact of such access is limited. The issue is a clinical as well as a legal one, and a number of important questions arise. Which patients want to see their records, and what psychodynamic issues may underlie the request? How and when are patients hurt by seeing their records? How and when do they benefit? How does patient access change what clinicians write in the chart, and what impact will such changes have on treatment?

Our search of the literature revealed only nine studies that have attempted to address these questions. Four reports involved medical patients, four were of psychiatric patients, and one bridged both groups by studying patients seen in consultation by psychiatrists during a medical or surgical hospitalization. The nine studies varied in quality.

Medical Patients. The four reports involving medical patients all reached favorable conclusions about patient access to records. Bouchard and others (1973) reported that outpatients receiving their records after initial evaluations generally felt reassured and less worried about their health. In a follow-up study at the same center, Bronson and others (1978) demonstrated further positive and no negative findings, although fewer patients appeared to be interested in record review than the researchers had expected.

In another investigation (Stevens and others, 1977), patients had to show some initiative in order to see the chart; surprisingly few asked for it. Only one research effort (Golodetz and others, 1976) attempted systematically to evaluate the impact on record-keeping practices. This effort found that, in 10 percent of the records, the physician modified content slightly, and in five instances he or she avoided psychiatric diagnoses altogether. Three of the four studies just cited were not controlled and provided the record to all patients; thus, they failed to discriminate the population that requests the chart and that may be at special risk of harm from the results of such a request.

Altman and others (1980) reviewed all psychiatric consultations on a medical and surgical service over a three-year period and identified sixteen patients who had read their charts on request. They then prospectively monitored six medical and surgical wards for six additional months and interviewed the eleven patients who asked to see their charts during that time. The patients in both groups were similar. Women outnumbered men by three to one, and all but one had a personality disorder. A higher than usual number had medically related jobs; many had chronic pain syndromes. All the patients were in conflict with staff at the time of their chart review request, and all the patients were seen as having compelling emotional needs. Nine of the ten patients diagnosed as having self-induced or factitious illness reacted angrily to their charts, and problems of ward management increased. In some cases, patient access to the chart was felt to decrease suspicion and to improve the patient's sense of control. The authors concluded that patients' requests to read their records were often symptomatic of an adversarial doctor–patient relationship and that such requests always exemplified mistrust.

Psychiatric Patients. Very little research addresses the impact of access to records on psychiatric inpatients or outpatients. One group of authors (Simonton and others, 1977; Stein and others, 1979) reported advantageous results when access to charts was provided in the presence of a staff member to all inpatients in a psychiatric unit over a five-month period. In follow-up questionnaires, the patients reported that they felt both better informed and more involved in their treatment, although they sometimes had been upset by what they had read. While the staff generally concluded that patient access to records had been therapeutic and that no substantial problems had developed from this practice, they also reported a number of ways in which the use of the chart underwent significant change. Fifty-eight percent of staff indicated that they did not record information likely to upset the patient. One third reported a new need to seek information from sources other than the chart. Twenty-six percent stated that they were less likely to diagnose a patient as psychotic because of open records. An independent review comparing the preaccess and access periods suggested that with open charting the staff had made more frequent notations of disruptive behavior and had more carefully corrected errors in the record. Although the impact on patients is reported to have been positive, the researchers made no attempt to control for access to the record. The staff remained generally favorably disposed toward open charting, yet the degree to which documentation habits changed raises important questions about the impact of open charting both on the record and on communications between staff.

McFarlane and others (1980) conducted a controlled study in which a cohort of psychiatric inpatients was advised of their right to see their records; 39 percent requested to do so. While a trend to feel better informed was noted among patients in this access group, statistical significance was not reached. There were no important differences in compliance with treatment, behavioral ratings, length of hospitalization, or attitudes toward hospital staff between these patients and those not allowed to read their records. No significant distinctions were noted by independent raters who compared nursing notes from the study and control groups. The majority of staff members reported feeling that they had made changes in recording practices. Most of these changes were improvements (for example, describing behavior more specifically). There were only two reports that less information had been included in the chart. These authors concluded that patient access to the chart can be therapeutic.

Bernstein and Andrews (1982) performed a retrospective chart review of those twenty-six inpatients who had requested to see their charts during a one-year period. Patients in this population were more likely to have character disorders, they tended to be younger, and they were often, albeit inferentially, considered to be responding to feelings of being misunderstood by staff.

In the only report including at least some psychiatric outpatients, Roth and others (1980) discussed a series of former inpatients and patients in ambulatory treatment who had made requests to see their records. During a period of eighteen months, sixteen requests were made. Four persons made no more than an initial inquiry. The twelve other persons were interviewed to learn their reasons for desiring the record. The sessions, including chart review when permitted, lasted between one and one and one half hours. Two of the twelve were denied access to the record completely, and in two other cases access was restricted to parts of the chart. The authors tentatively concluded that patients are not likely to be harmed by reading their records and they may even benefit. Their conclusions must be viewed in the context of a strictly controlled right of access, including careful screening by a hospital administrator, who seems to have devoted a considerable amount of time to each request. Further, fully one third of the patients were in fact restricted from at least some portion of the chart.

The research done so far illuminates a number of interesting points. To begin with, most studies reported that fewer patients than expected showed an interest in seeing their charts, especially when patients had to initiate the process themselves. There is no evidence that, if access laws become universal, public interest would generate an unwieldy demand. One author (O'Gara, 1984) has hypothesized that curiosity may even decline. There are no known instances of malpractice suits stemming from a patient's access to his or her record, and many professionals believe that record review may improve interactions between patients and staff. Although the studies summarized here generally concluded that seeing the chart was beneficial to patients, the results are at least somewhat contradictory with reference to psychiatric patients, and they do demonstrate some potential pitfalls.

The Function of the Record, Privacy, and Informed Consent

It may be that reading his or her medical record often leaves the patient feeling better informed. It may even be that mistrust is diminished and the physician–patient relationship is enhanced, although surely there are important exceptions. The question remains, Should the patient's record be used for these purposes? Advocates of patients' legal rights contend that the wish to withhold the record stems from the paternalism (Felch, 1976) and the mystification (Kaiser, 1975) inherent in the practice of medicine. They argue that, if reviewing the record may enhance patient autonomy, the practice should be implemented without question. Medical and mental health practitioners counter that these premises belie a fundamental misunderstanding of the purpose of record keeping. Clinicians have used the chart as a valuable working tool. It serves as a medium of communication between colleagues and staff, and it was never intended to be meaningful to the patient. The practitioner's responsibility to keep his or her patient well informed has been seen as an issue quite distinct from the keeping of charts, especially in the area of mental health.

Our scrutiny of the existing research gives us reason to believe that the use of medical and mental health records as uncensored communications between professionals may change if patients have access to records. The recording of psychodynamic material, especially of the therapist's speculations, will be greatly affected. Projective psychological test reporting is perhaps the most vivid example of inferential data that the patient would have a hard time understanding; at the worst, reading such data could be emotionally damaging. It is questionable whether such material can be written in a fashion suitable for patient review without seriously compromising its value to other professionals (Smith, 1978).

The strongest arguments for the right of medical and psychiatric patients to have access to their own records stem from the right to privacy and from the necessity for informed consent for the release of records. Denial of the right to review one's record may seriously abridge a patient's ability to assert and protect his or her personal privacy (Kaiser, 1975). Patients are constantly asked to give their consent to the disclosure of information from their records. It may be impossible to obtain third-party reimbursements without such a release. Truly informed consent to this type of request may be contingent on patients' being familiar with the material in the record. Without knowledge of the actual contents, patients are asked to reveal information about themselves that will enter large data banks, where it will forever be beyond their control, without their having verified it for accuracy. Surely, consent for such divulgence cannot be informed if the patient does not have access to the record.

Traditional standards of confidentiality are being threatened, much as other societal trends are changing time-honored concepts of the doctor–patient relationship and patient autonomy. The growth of statutory rights of access to personal records has occurred partially in response to the dangers of enlarging pools of information maintained on individuals in all areas of our lives. Medical and mental health records are merely the latest examples.

Requirements for Safe Access Statutes: Ten Recommendations

As increasing numbers of access laws are presented in state legislatures, it would seem incumbent on clinicians to advocate for their patients by supporting those bills that provide for access in the safest possible manner. Opposing such legislation on purely speculative grounds without an empirical base seems particularly futile. Case-by-case litigation is less methodical, and it can produce anomalous results. In one case, the decision to make records available was based on whether the hospital received state aid in the form of legislative appropriations (Nokes, 1978); in another, it was based on whether the hospital was a public agency generating public records (Madden, 1982).

Our work leads us to a number of conclusions about the requirements for such statutes. If a right to read one's record is to be established, it must be qualified in order to protect a number of competing interests, including the patient's well-being, the patient's ongoing treatment, the privacy and confidentiality of third parties, the special needs of minors, and the ability of health practitioners to keep notes for their own use. The recommendations that we present are specifically applicable to psychiatric records. The order in which we present them says nothing about their relative importance.

First, access laws must contain exceptions allowing for the withholding of records when the practitioner believes that the patient will be harmed by viewing them. The definition of harm should be broad and not limited to predictions of self-destructive or assaultive behavior. If the practitioner's decision is contested, the patient should have a right to appeal to someone who has the authority to release. We urge that such independent review should be conducted in organized care facilities by the medical director, chief of psychiatry, or other similarly situated individual. Provisions for mediating refusals to private outpatients should preferably be made through professional peer review mechanisms or perhaps through state agencies. Beyond this nonadversarial step, patients should be entitled to petition for judicial review and determination in each case.

Second, the review of records should be at the patient's own risk, and treatment personnel should not be held responsible for unforeseen harm that may result. Of course, clinicians should be expected to make reasonable efforts to protect the patient.

Third, in order to assess the risk-benefit ratio, a practitioner must be entitled to ask the patient his or her reason for seeking access. Such requests may reflect discord within the therapeutic relationship, and discussion may allow for the resolution of such conflicts.

Fourth, a reasonable period of time should be allowed for complying with the request—one long enough to allow the practitioner to produce and review the record and discuss the request but short enough to conform to the intent of due process.

Fifth, while access to the record should be at reasonable cost to the patient, a means of reimbursement for the time that the clinician devotes to the process must be established. The argument that record sharing is an important tool of patient education and thus therapeutic could be one basis for requiring third-party payment.

Sixth, while we strongly believe that reading the record in the presence of the clinician will facilitate the patient's comprehension, we wonder how this could effectively be required for former patients, particularly those who are disgruntled. Those presently under care should review the record in the presence of the primary therapist or some other qualified staff member.

Seventh, access statutes should require the consent of minors above a specified age, perhaps twelve to fourteen years, before their records are provided to their parents.

Eighth, given the sensitive nature of information often supplied only by family members, friends, or other third parties, laws should provide for the deletion of such material at the clinician's discretion. Such stipulations will protect both the confidentiality of third parties and the integrity of charting practices that require the inclusion of such information in order to record the patient's history accurately.

Ninth, access statutes should specifically permit the keeping of personal notes, in any and all treatment settings, that are not accessible to the patient. This provision may be especially critical for exploratory psychotherapies, wherein process notes and psychodynamic speculations are vital to the conduct of therapy and supervision. They are in no way crucial to the patient.

Last, patients should have only a limited right to alter the record. The clinician may revise the record at the patient's request when he or she agrees that there is a factual error. Although this position may be controversial, it is our view that, if the patient feels that the record contains inaccurate or incomplete information and if the practitioner will not correct it, the patient should be able to place his or her own addendum permanently in the chart.

The evidence is far from in regarding the impact that access laws will have, especially for outpatients. While we would certainly like to know more before instituting any change that may influence the care of patients, the societal pressures promoting increased patient access to medical records are unlikely to decelerate in the interest of research. Psychiatrists and other clinicians can minimize any potential for harm accompanying the establishment of this nascent right by playing an active role in the political process of shaping appropriate legislation. As the data continue to evolve, amendments reflecting this improved understanding should be introduced, and the results should be evaluated scientifically.

References

Altman, J. H., Reich, P., Kelly, M. J., and Rogers, M. P. "Patients Who Read Their Hospital Charts." *New England Journal of Medicine,* 1980, *302,* 169–171.

American Psychiatric Association. "Model Law on Confidentiality of Health and Social Service Records." *American Journal of Psychiatry,* 1979, *136,* 138–144.

Anthony, M. F. "Issues Relating to Patients' Access to Their Medical Records." *Medical Record News,* 1977, *48* (6), 85–91.

Bernstein, R. A., and Andrews, E. M. "Response Strategies for Chart Requests from Psychiatric Inpatients." *Hospital and Community Psychiatry,* 1982, *33,* 841–843.

Bouchard, R. E., Tufo, H. M., Van Buren, H. C., Eddy, W. M., Twitchell, J. C., and Bedard, L. "The Patient and His Problem-Oriented Medical Record." In H. K. Walker, J. W. Hurst, and M. F. Woody (Eds.), *Applying the Problem-Oriented System.* New York: Medcom Press, 1973.

Bronson, D. L., Rubin, A. S., and Tufo, H. M. "Patient Education Through Record Sharing." *Quality Review Bulletin,* 1978, *4* (12), 2–4.

California Health and Safety Code, Division 20, Chapter 6.7, Sections 25250–25258. *West Cumulative Pocket Part,* 1984.

Felch, E. "Access to Medical and Psychiatric Records: Proposed Legislation." *Albany Law Review,* 1976, *40,* 580–617.

Golodetz, A., Ruess, J., and Milhous, R. L. "The Right to Know: Giving the Patient His Medical Record." *Archives of Physical Medicine and Rehabilitation,* 1976, *57,* 78–81.

Gotkin v. *Miller,* 379 F. Supp. 859 (E.D. N.Y. 1974) *aff'd* 514 F.2d 125 (2d Cir. 1975).

Kaiser, B. L. "Patients' Rights of Access to Their Own Medical Records: The Need for New Law." *Buffalo Law Review,* 1975, *24,* 317–330.

McFarlane, W. J. G., Bowman, R. H., and MacInnes, M. "Patient Access to Hospital Records: A Pilot Project." *Canadian Journal of Psychiatry,* 1980, *25,* 497–502.

Madden, J. M. "Patient Access to Medical Records in Washington." *Washington Law Review,* 1982, *57,* 697–713.

Nokes, G. B. "Patient's Right of Access Limited to Records of Hospitals Receiving Legislative Appropriations: *Doe v. Institute of Living, Inc.*" *Connecticut Law Review,* 1978, *11,* 44–61.

O'Gara, S. "Does Patient Access to Health Records Cause Harm? A Review of the Literature." *Journal of the American Medical Record Association,* 1984, *55* (3), 20–22.

Roth, L. H., Wolford, J., and Meisel, A. "Patient Access to Records: Tonic or Toxin?" *American Journal of Psychiatry,* 1980, *137,* 592–596.

Simonton, M. H., Neuffer, C. H., Stein, E. J., and Furedy, R. L. "The Open Medical Record: An Educational Tool." *Journal of Psychiatric Nursing and Mental Health Services,* 1977, *15* (12), 25–30.

Smith, W. H. "Ethical, Social, and Professional Issues in Patients' Access to Psychological Test Reports." *Bulletin of the Menninger Clinic,* 1978, *42,* 150–155.

Stein, E. J., Furedy, R. L., Simonton, M. J., and Neuffer, C. H. "Patient Access to Medical Records on a Psychiatric Inpatient Unit." *American Journal of Psychiatry,* 1979, *136,* 327–329.

Stevens, D. P., Stagg, R., and MacKay, I. R. "What Happens When Hospitalized Patients See Their Own Records?" *Annals of Internal Medicine,* 1977, *86,* 474–477.

Tucker, G. "Patient Access to Medical Records." *Legal Aspects of Medical Practice,* 1978, *6* (10), 45–50.

U.S. Department of Health, Education, and Welfare. *Report of the Secretary's Commission on Medical Malpractice.* DHEW Publication No. (OS) 73–88. Washington, D.C.: U.S. Department of Health, Education, and Welfare, 1973.

*Harold I. Schwartz is a physician-in-charge, psychiatric inpatient
service, Beth Israel Medical Center, New York, and assistant
professor of clinical psychiatry, Mount Sinai School of Medicine.*

*Stephen Rachlin is chairman, Department of Psychiatry and
Psychology, Nassau County Medical Center (East Meadow, New
York); associate professor of clinical psychiatry, State University of
New York at Stony Brook School of Medicine; and special professor
of law and psychiatry, Hofstra University School of Law.*

*This postscript outlines several points to consider in examining
the issues presented in the preceding chapters.*

Conclusions

Stephen Rachlin

Having begun my opening notes with a question, let me do the same in this
denouement: How does one synthesize all the material gathered in the preceding pages, and to what end? Clearly, some of the authors have been more stri-
dent than others, but there are some problems inherently more troublesome to
us. The traditions of our professional lives, particularly our fiercely protected
independence, are giving way to social necessity. Demands of the times in
which we now function could not have been anticipated by our predecessors,
leaving us less than completely prepared to deal with the "surprises" that are
now facts unlikely to go away quietly. It is certain that some beneficial modifications have resulted from judicial and legislative activism.

Many of the changes imposed on psychiatric practice have initially
been met with broad opposition from clinicians. Often, this evolves relatively
rapidly into considering appropriate limitations of new or novel proposals,
under what conditions postulated "rights" should be granted, and details of
their administration. While the righteousness of all of this may in the final
estimate be a matter of philosophy, our patients will derive the greatest gain
from scientific scrutiny of how far it all goes toward meeting their needs.

Those of us who, in one or another capacity, are or have been involved
in teaching legal professionals (and most of the contributors to this sourcebook
so qualify) are well aware that simple polemicism leads nowhere other than
perhaps further polarization. Despite this caveat, it can serve a valuable didactic
purpose in sensitizing the nonspecialist to multifaceted concerns and questions.

S. Rachlin (Ed.). *Legal Encroachment on Psychiatric Practice.* New Directions for
Mental Health Services, no. 25. San Francisco: Jossey-Bass, March 1985.

I hope that the foregoing chapters have been a spring board for thought, since it is the ultimate responsibility of us all to exert our influence and knowledge as to what is clinically most reasonable on those who write and interpret the laws under which we operate.

Stephen Rachlin is chairman, Department of Psychiatry and Psychology, Nassau County Medical Center (East Meadow, New York); associate professor of clinical psychiatry, State University of New York at Stony Brook School of Medicine; and special professor of law and psychiatry, Hofstra University School of Law.

Index